Conservation and Management of Indigenous Breeds of Cattle for Sustainable Utilization

Dr. B.L. Pander
Ex. Professor & Head
Department of Animal Genetics and Breeding
LUVAS, Hisar-125 004

Dr. Ravindra Sharma
Ex Director research
LUVAS, Hisar-125 004

Dr. D. S. Dalal
Professor
Department of Animal Genetics and Breeding
LUVAS, Hisar-125 004

Dr. Ankit Magotra
Assistant Professor
Department of Animal Genetics and Breeding
LUVAS, Hisar-125 004

SATISH SERIAL PUBLISHING HOUSE
403, Express Tower, Commercial Complex
Azadpur, Delhi-110033 (India)
Phone : 011-27672852, Fax : 91-11-27672046
e-mail : info@satishserial.com, hkjain1975@yahoo.com
Website : www.satishserial.com

Published by :

SATISH SERIAL PUBLISHING HOUSE
403, Express Tower, Commercial Complex, Azadpur, Delhi-110033 (INDIA)
Phone : 011-27672852 Fax : 91-11-27672046
E-mail : info@satishserial.com, hkjain1975@yahoo.com

ISBN 978-93-86200-43-3

Composed, Designed & Printed in India

Dedicated

to

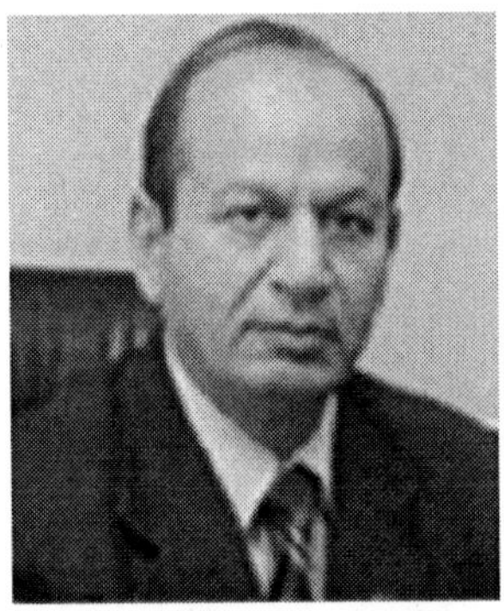

Maj Gen Shri Kant, SM, VSM (Retd)

President, National Academy of Veterinary Sciences (India)
Former Vice-Chancellor, LUVAS, Hisar

Foreword

Our Indigenous cattle breeds which are the humped cattle, are thought to be the world's oldest domesticated cattle. Cow has been a foundation of Indian agriculture for centuries and has served as source of nutrition for farmer's families through milk and milk products, as well as providing draught animal power for both agricultural operations such as ploughing and tilling the land, as well as for transportation of goods. However, mechanization, crossbreeding and low productivity leads to extinction of our valuable germplasm. Thus, there is an urgent need to conserve, improve and propagate our valuable germplasm. I am very much confident that the present book is a commendable contribution with complete information in this direction. I, therefore feel extreme sense of happiness in writing the foreword for this book entitled *"Conservation and Management of Indigenous Breeds of Cattle for Sustainable Utilization"* and express gratitude to the authors team for compiling such a valuable information. I sincerely hope that the report will be useful to all stakeholders, for planning and policy making purposes and also for research and academic purposes.

Dr. Gurdial Singh
Vice-Chancellor
LUVAS, Hisar (Haryana)

Preface

India has a very rich reservoir of genetic diversity and possesses some of the best breeds of cattle in the world. The native livestock breeds exhibit a distinct superiority in utilization of poor quality feed and are well adapted to hot and humid climate and resistant to tropical diseases. Genetic variation in animals has developed over millions of years. In the course of time the usefulness of different genes and gene combinations has been under severe tests, especially concerning adaptability to different conditions and resistance to diseases and parasites. Compared to 18th Livestock Census 2007, the indigenous cattle population has decreased by 8.94 per cent and crossbred population increased by 20.18 per cent. The population of cattle decreased by 3.14 per cent in rural and 18.34 per cent in urban areas. Thus, there is an urgent need to conserve, improve and propagate our important indigenous cattle breeds.

The present book entitled *"Conservation and Management of Indigenous Breeds of Cattle for Sustainable Utilization"* presents the current status, problems and conservation strategies of our valuable indigenous cattle breeds at institute, state and national level. The suggested programmes and policies are an outcome of the deliberations among members of the working groups and the regional consultations with stakeholders in livestock development. The subject matter has been collected and compiled from various books, journals and web sources, arranged and expressed in simple language as per requirement of the students, researchers and policy makers. I thank authors and other participants for their valuable inputs. I hope the suggestions and strategies contained in this book will serve an important input for developing effective policies and implementable programmes at field level.

Authors

Contents

Executive Summary

Livestock plays a vital role in the economic development of an country where 70 per cent population is dependent on Agriculture. In India, 24.8 per cent of the agricultural GDP was contributed by Livestock sector and with national GDP contribution 3.9 per cent during 2013-14. At present, the total milk production of India is 146 million tons, cattle contributes 45 per cent in total milk production i.e. 61.65 million tons (Exotic/crossbred 29.5 per cent and zebu/non-descript 25.4 per cent) making India a leader in terms of highest milk production in the world. The increased production of milk has improved the per capita availability to 337 g/day but it still remains half the world average. The major concern of country is the low productivity of indigenous animals and huge dairy losses due to production related diseases in high yielding cattle.

The total cattle population is 190.90 millions out of which indigenous cattle population is 151.17 millions and exotic/crossbred is 39.73 millions (19th Livestock census, 2012). Compared to 18th Livestock census, 2007 the total indigenous cattle population decreased by 8.94per cent and exotic crossbred population increased by 20.18 per cent. The population of cattle decreased by 3.14 per cent in rural and 18.34 per cent in urban areas. Thus, there is an urgent need to conserve, improve and propagate our important indigenous cattle breed Prior to formulation of any strategy for the improvement of these breeds we need to understand why we should promote indigenous breeds? The reasons for adoption of such breeds are following:

Indigenous cattle are

i) Robust and resilent

ii) Particularly suited to the climate and environment of their respective breeding tracts.

iii) Endowed with qualities of heat tolerance,

iv) Resistant to diseases

v) Capable of producing under low plane of nutrition

vi) Playing vital role in rural festivals and rituals.

vii) Producing milk and other products (panchgavya) which are beneficial for human health.

The salient recommendations are as follows

Conservation of our natural biodiversity and genetic pool is essential as these breeds are essentially the products of long term natural and artificial selection and are better adapted to regional fodder, environment and perform under low and medium inputs. Such utility genes and gene pools should be identified, conserved and utilized for breeding and research, particularly in the era of climate change.

These indigenous breeds are mostly reared among small and marginal farmers who keep 1-2 animals to meet out their own requirements only and not for commercial purposes.

The reasons/constrains for erosion of indigenous breeds may be divided into two major categories:

a) **Intrinsic factors:** Low genetic potential for production.

b) **Extrinsic factors:** Poor nutrition/feed management, inferior farm practices, ineffective veterinary and extension services, inefficient implementation of breed improvement programmes, non-availability of quality males for breeding.

A. Strategies for conservation and development of indigenous cattle

a) National level

i) **Development of a centralized online database management system** which is very much essential now days. In case of indigenous cattle there is no adequate and efficient data base management system in India.

ii) It is proposed to establish **indigenous cattle breed parks** in different states. Breed parks will serve as: **Education hubs and Tourist spot.**

iii) **Indi Cattle Card (ICC):** Breed wise unqiue identification number must be allotted to indigenous cattle to overcome problems of indiscriminate breeding, breed dilution and unauthentic data.

iv) **It is proposed to set up an INTRABULL (common progeny testing between different states)** programme at national level on Sahiwal, Gir, Tharparkar, Hariana and other important indigenous cattle breeds involving farmers.There should be a single genetic improvement programme for each important breed at national level. Breeds which are economically viable and are accepted by the common farmers, should be conserved through *In-situ* conservation using ONBS with MOET model involving large population throughout the breeding tract. Better synchronization and convergence in the research efforts of various research and development Institutions including the ICAR, SAU and SVU, All India Coordinated Research Projects, National Bureaus, NGOs and private sector R&D institutions will be necessary for optimum utilization of research resources and efforts.

v) There is an urgent need to restructure and strengthen infrastructure of veterinary institutions, vaccine and diagnostic production units, indigenous cattle breeds semen stations and artificial insemination breeding farms, feed and fodder production units, etc. for effective utilization and for ensuring optimal services. The Government will create enabling environment at the national level and inclusive planning at regional and community level for generation and delivery of these services in the rural and urban areas.

vi) **National Breeding policy:** Crossbreeding with exotic strains should be totally banned in the home tracts of the important indigenous cattle breeds. Identify the geographical boundaries of the areas where non-descript cattle should be upgraded by crossing with bulls of indigenous breeds. Once such areas are earmarked, no cross-breeding of non-descript cattle, other than with bulls of indigenous breeds, should be permitted. This measure will provide an incentive to the farmers in the breeding tracts to rear male stock of indigenous breeds up to the breeding age, as the demand will create a market for the bull semen or natural service. Consequently, the practice of disposing off the male calves will be curbed to some extents.

vii) **Rediscovering properties of Panchgavya** with well planned research experiments.

viii) **Publication and patenting** of important findings on indigenous cow milk, urine, dung.

ix) **New breeding and reproductive technologies**, developed from time to time, will be adopted for faster implementation of various breed improvement programmes and for increasing production and propagation.

x) **Semen sexing technology:** Efforts should be made to develop **indigenous semen sexing technology** to provide greater choice regarding breeding to farmers. The delivery of breeding services would be regulated by fixing standards with periodic evaluation of service providers.

xi) **Marketing facilities for indigenous cow milk, milk products and byproducts**:

Marketing facility is inadequate and often unorganized. Lack of proper marketing facility and related infrastructure demoralize our animal keepers. It is necessary to create necessary infrastructure, policy and procedures to organize animal trade for better returns to farmers and faster growth of livestock sector.

b) State Level

i) Re-orientation of Breeding Policy for indigenous cattle:

Selective breeding of defined indigenous breeds of cattle having high milk yield, and those with excellent draught abilities, will be promoted to improve their production and reproduction potential. This will help in propagation, conservation and genetic upgradation. Production of breeding bulls having high genetic potential will be an essential element of the breeding policy and breed.

Formation of breed associations by involving farmers for improvement of indigenous breeds of cattle and online registration of animals having good genetic potential would be promoted by providing financial, technical and organizational assistance.

ii) **SAU / SVU / Institutional herds mandate:** Breeds which no longer find favour with the farmers and are near to extinction, whatever the reason, should be identified and these breeds should be preserved only in the institutional farms with improved conservation technologies.

iii) Multiplication of elite animals by using various reproductive biotechnologies like MOET and Cloning.

iv) **Use of stray cattle** with normal reproduction as a foster mothers in Embryo transfer programmes.

v) Establishment of government certified Semen banks of indigenous breeds and facility for A.I at farmers door step.

vi) **Syllabus:** Creation of interest among young generation via introduction of practical courses in state board examinations and must visit to various organized farms and gaushalas as a compuslary mandate in the syllabus.

vii) **Women empowerment** by linking them with Gau Samvardhen and organic farming.

viii) **Linking to ayurhubs (Patanjali, Dabur etc):** There is an urgent need to establish dung and urine collection centres at various places linked to ayurhubs (Pitanjali, Dabur etc).

ix) Establishing sale counters as a part of marketing strategies for milk and milk products of indigenous cattle (**A2 + Organic Milk**).

x) **Capacity building** through education, training, awareness and information sharing.

c) Regional Level

i) **Involvement of local communities and institutions** in the design, implementation and ownership of breeding strategies.

ii) **Incentives to farmers:** Encouraging farmers by giving incentives for keeping high producing indigenous animals and purchasing males from them on premium.

iii) Rearing of males in various clusters and distributing them to village panchayats/poor farmers on subsidized rates.

iv) **Setting up of animal feed and mineral mixture manufacturing units** in a clusters of villages by farmer groups.

v) Setting up of milk products manufacturing and pasteurization units in each cluster by farmer groups.

- **Strengthening cooperative chain** especially for indigenous cow milk, dung and urine at regional level. Services must be provided at farmers door step i.e daily collection of milk, dung and urine at set price for encouraging farmers to keep even non-lactating animals.
- **Promotion of organic cattle farming** for the welfare of animals and promoting human and soil health.
- **Bull / semen certification agency**: It is proposed to set up bull/semen certification agency. At present bulls used in villages/ gaushalas / panchyats are not certified that leads to serious consequences viz., breed dilution and reduced production.

B. Strategies for enhancement of milk production in indigenous cattle

Efforts for promoting indigenous breeds must be undertaken in two different directions and on the basis of type of livestock owner i.e different routes of strategies must be formulated, one targeting small and marginal farmers and second targeting commercial dairy farmers. Greatest potential for improvement resides in small and marginal farmers which are on low Milk production systems.

A brief outline of different approaches which can be followed aiming for enhancement of milk production in indigenous breeds is given below:

a) Breeding initiatives

i) Milk production is a sex-limited trait and hence need a programme for intense and accurate selection of males of these indigenous breeds. Seventy five per cent genetic improvement in milk production comes through selection of males which requires extensive Artificial Insemination and performance recording network. For example: North America and Europe have doubled milk production potential by efficient large scale progeny testing programme. But, policies of these countries may not be applicable as such to our country, where most of the farmers keep 1-2 animals. Despite of vigorous Govt. initiatives for crossbreeding and Murrah buffalo improvement programmes. AI services cover only 25 per cent of dairy animals, therefore, it will be our mistake to neglect upgradation of indigenous breeds through natural service.

ii) Therefore, optimum number of superior quality breeding bulls of good and proved genetic merits are to be used through both A.I. and natural mating. Such bulls may be provided to village Panchayats with provision of manpower and funds to keep them.

iii) Brazil has demonstrated that it is possible to get a gain of 1per cent of phenotypic mean per year in lactation yield of Indian Zebu cattle. They have successfully implemented progeny testing and Open Nucleus Breeding System (ONBS) with MOET for Gir, Kanrej, Ongole, Sindhi and Kangayam breeds of cattle imported from India, itself. This example represents success and applicability of such programmes for these breeds.

iv) Presently progeny testing programme for Sahiwal and Gir (by CIRC) is going on which is a small programme as it involves less than 2per cent population and testing of 10-20 bulls per year only. Such programmes may be initiated for other breeds also with wholly operational mode not to be implemented in Institiutional herds only but involving rural farmers also.

v) **Extensive castration Programme-** Males of non-descript breeds and or used for drought purpose should be castrated. Concerned A.H. Deptt./Agricultural/Veterinary University/NGOs may take initiatives for such programme in states, taking up village/ block one by one.

vi) Further, prior to formulation of any breeding policy at national/ state level, it must be considered that promotion of any breed must not be done to the extent such that it may pose threat to other breeds. Murrah initiatives programmes in Haryana certainly toss up population and production of Murrah buffalo in the state have neglected Hariana breed of cattle as a result its population is in decreasing phase.

vii) Immediate survey of all indigenous breeds may be done prior to formulation of any breeding strategy.

b) Feeding management

i) As for all cattle/bovine/livestock assets, availability and quality of feed and fodder is increasingly becoming a challenge. The current deficit of green fodder and concentrate is reported to be 34 per cent. Hence, we can't assume for higher/improved production without subsiding this challenge.

ii) Further, imbalanced nutrition is major factor responsible for low livestock production and other problems like – higher age at first calving and longer inter-calving period, anestrous and other reproductive problems which may lead to non-adoptability of indigenous breeds especially, as feed supplementation / mineral mixture feeding is being done at commercial farms with crossbred animals but is not practised by small farmers rearing indigenous breeds which further mould the scenario.

iii) Therefore, balanced feed requirements must be re-formulated keeping in view regional availability of feed and fodders and specific requirements of indigenous breeds. Standards must be developed for compound feed for such breeds giving locally available ingredients priority.

iv) Blood biochemical profiling of these breeds may be taken locally/ regionally to know the actual picture as which minerals are deficient in these breeds and to be compared with soil and green fodder profile.

v) Regulating Authority for Livestock feed/Monitoring quality of livestock feed: States may collect random samples of different brands/unbranded commercial livestock feeds sold in market and test accordance with BIS standards.

c) Extension services

Effective implementation and delivery of improvement programmes to grass root farmers is mandatory, which necessitates the effective livestock extension network for delivery of technical expertise for improving milk production in these indigenous cattle breeds. Currently, less than 1per cent of the total plan budget for the animal husbandry sector is allocated for extension activities. This must be increased substantially as the sector which needs most attention is neglected most till date. Further, progressive farmers also need to be trained to act as extension agents for disseminating technical knowledge.

Knowledge gap: Most of the livestock producers being small and marginal farmers, their capacity to mobilize resources required to absorb the latest technologies developed by research institutions are limited. Absence of effective extension machinery for this purpose compounds the problem. Lack of access to institutional finance is a major constraint in attracting investment required for improving productivity by adopting latest technology.

❑❑❑

CHAPTER-1

Introduction

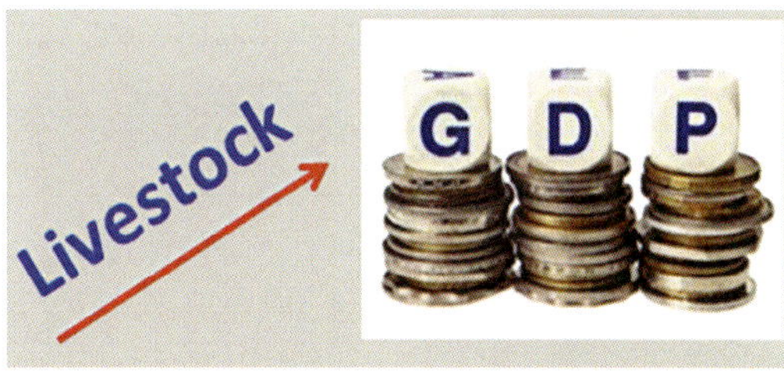

Livestock inputs and outputs are growing economic sectors. More than a billion people in Asia keep livestock, 60 per cent of rural households do so. It is the major income source of the poor and especially of women in developing countries. Livestock is an integral part of India's agricultural economy and plays a multifaceted role in providing livelihood support to the rural population. The dairy industry in particular, plays a strong role for the livelihood of poor people because agriculture land is shrinking due to fast urbanization and as a result dependency of farmers is increasing on dairy sector.

Animal production is the backbone of agriculture sector as also in the economic and social development of our country. Having passed through an era of green revolution, the growth in agricultural production has slowed down, while the growth in animal production is still keeping up at encouraging pace. This is the highly concerned and neglected sector where the poor contributes to growth directly instead of getting benefit from growth generated elsewhere.

The overall growth rate in livestock sector is steady and is around 4-5 per cent and this has been achieved despite the fact that investment in this sector was not substantial. The growth in the sector results in reasonable development of the rural economy particularly in reducing the poverty amongst the weaker sections. The rural women are directly involved in most of the operations relating to animal farming and play a significant role in Animal Husbandry.

1.1 Role of livestock sector in agricultural economy

Livestock sector is an important sub-sector of the agriculture of Indian economy. The livestock production and agriculture are interdependent and intrinsically linked, playing a crucial role for the overall food security. Livestock plays a vital role in the economic development. In India, during 2013-14, 24.8 per cent of the agricultural GDP was contributed by this sector and contribution of this sector to national GDP was 3.9 per cent.

According to Central Statistics Office (CSO) estimates, gross domestic product from livestock sector was about Rs. 507 billion during 1993-94 (accounting for 22.86per cent of agriculture and allied GDP).This rose to Rs. 4060 billion during 2013-14 with 24.8per cent share in the agriculture and allied sector. The growth in agriculture sector over the years has been steady and fluctuating significantly depending upon the monsoon and other climatic factors. Of late there has been deceleration of agricultural growth. Livestock sector on the contrary has shown a steady growth and thus providing stability to the overall family income.

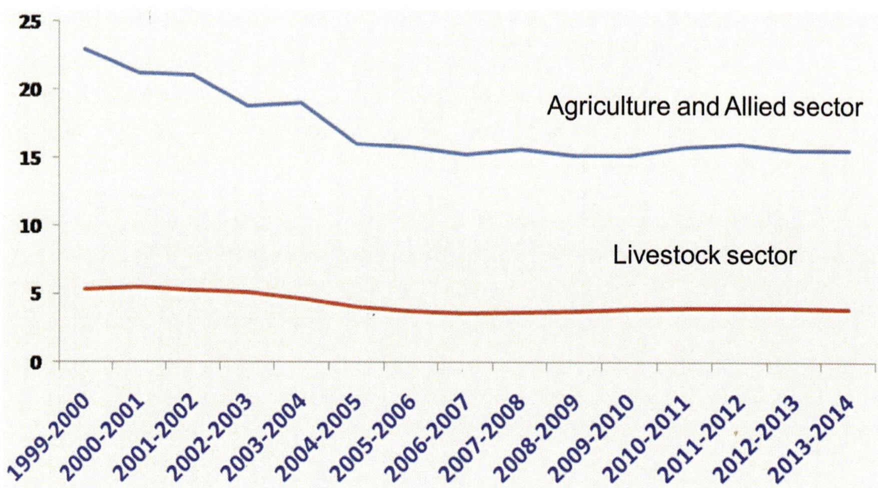

Figure 1.1 Contribution of livestock and Agriculture in GDP

Table 1.1 Percentage contribution of livestock sector to agriculture and national GDP (at 2004-2005 prices).

Year	Per cent Contribution of Livestock sector to	
	Agriculture GDP	National GDP
1999-2000	23.12	5.30
2000-2001	25.61	5.44
2001-2002	24.69	5.21
2002-2003	27.00	5.08
2003-2004	24.49	4.66
2004-2005	25.04	4.02
2005-2006	23.75	3.76
2006-2007	23.60	3.61
2007-2008	23.64	3.69
2008-2009	24.85	3.78
2009-2010	25.53	3.88
2010-2011	24.99	3.94
2011-2012*	24.70	4.00
2012-2013*	25.40	4.00
2013-2014*	15.60	3.90

* At 2011-2012 prices

❑❑❑

CHAPTER-2

Cattle Population Trend

The 19th livestock census showed an overall decline of 3.33 per cent in the total livestock population as compared to the previous census of 2007. As per the census data, cattle population has declined by 4 per cent to 1.90 crore in 2012 from 1.99 crore in 2007. The indigenous cattle population decreased by 8.94 per cent and crossbred population increased by 20.18 per cent. The population of cattle decreased by 3.14 per cent in rural and 18.34 per cent in urban areas.

Some of the states are truly regarded as a hub of dairy contributors to the national pool because of excellent dairy breeds of cattle. Haryana is blessed with some of the best breeds of the country. As per Livestock Census-2012, livestock population of the State is 88.19 lakh including 18.08 lakh cattle and 60.85 lakh buffaloes. The crossbred cattle strength has increased tremendously (75.92 per cent) whereas the indigenous cattle strength has gone down with a negative growth of 17.66per cent compared to last census which alarms for the conservation of a few important breeds for the present time and the time to come.

Thus, there is an urgent need to conserve, improve and propagate our important indigenous cattle breeds.

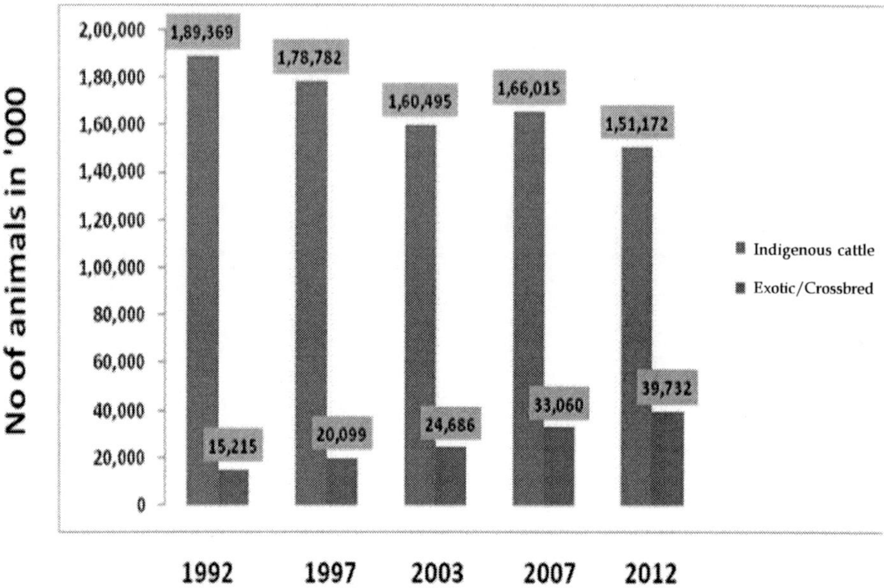

Figure 2.1 Indigenous and crossbred/ exotic population during 1992-2012.

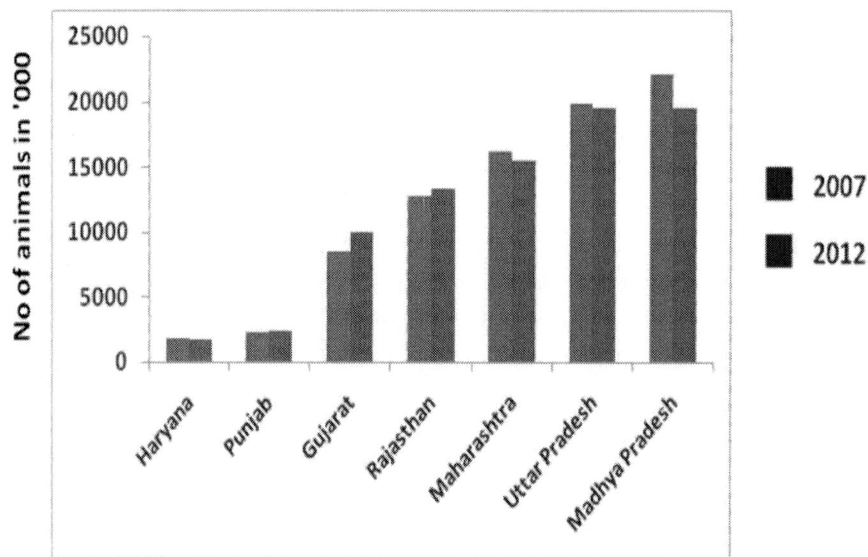

Figure 2.2 Comparative indigenous/non descript cattle population statistics in Haryana and neighboring states (2007-2012).

Table 1.2 Indigenous/Non-descript cattle population in Haryana and neighbouring states.

States/UTs	2007	2012
Haryana	1822.37	1808.12
Punjab	2322.29	2427.71
Gujarat	8567.7	9983.95
Rajasthan	12800.34	13324.46
Maharashtra	16268.25	15484.21
Uttar Pradesh	19885.45	19557.07
Madhya Pradesh	22121.79	19602.37

As shown in Figure 2.2 Indigenous/non-descript population is decreasing. The surprising fact is that the places where the declining trend is prominent now-a-days, were once the breeding tracks of world famous indigenous breeds of cattle. Furthermore, the animals which are existing in the field are not true to the breed; their germplasm is diluted by indiscriminate breeding.

This alarming situation needs to be critically evaluated for understanding the cause of the problem. Further, steps has to be taken to promote the indigenous cattle population in rural households so that the conservation efforts will be successful.

2.1 Stray cattle population

Stray cattle roaming around freely in the cities have become a serious menace. The root cause of the problem is the unplanned dairies, inside and around various cities. **The owners, after milking the cattle, leave them loose so that they can graze outside. Non-milking cattle are also left loose to save on their feed.**

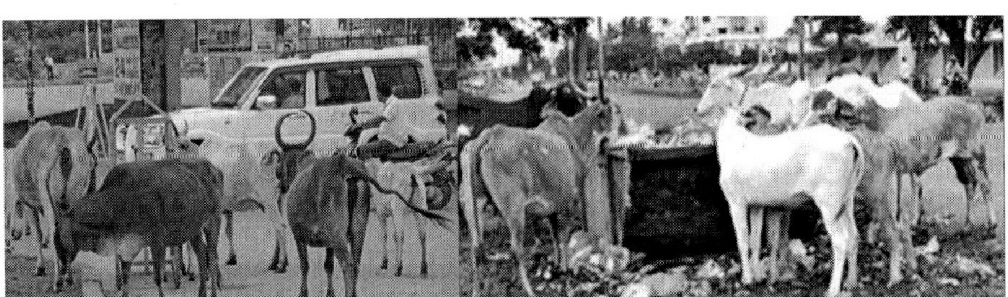

As per 19th Livestock Census, (2012), total stray cattle population is 52.87 lakh. This is a burning and serious problem in almost all states of India. Figure 2.3 representing number of stray cattle in Haryana and neighboring states. Comparative statistics (Figure 2.3 and 2.4) show density of stray cattle is highest in Uttar Pradesh followed by Rajasthan than Haryana.

The problems of impounding these cattle are many:

a) The paucit of trained man power with the municipal corporations.

b) Lack of gaushalas with adequate space.

c) Lack of cooperation from the society.

d) No legal framework.

In order to combat this problem; few recommendations are as follows :

a) Castration of young males

b) The authorities have to create large number of gaushalas, at appropriate locations, which can house thousands of such cattle.

c) Link stray animal protection and conservation project with Swachh Bharat Abhiyaný, keeping in mind their welfare as these animals depend upon garbage and polythene that leads to serious health disorders.

d) legal framework that municipal corporation has to take it as project i.e impounded cattle, should be released only with a fine of minimum Rs 5,000 per animal. The revenue raised can be used to maintain the cattle pounds and also pay for the cattle catchers. There should also be regular auctions of these cattle so that it fetches revenue, and also eases pressure on the pounds.

e) Contractual tenders half yearly basis to maintain stray cattle linked to various ayurhubs for urine and dung collection. Revenue generated used to maintain the cattle and payment of contractual labours.

f) Stray cattle cess like education cess.

g) Extra point tickets to mobilize revenue for Gaushalas.

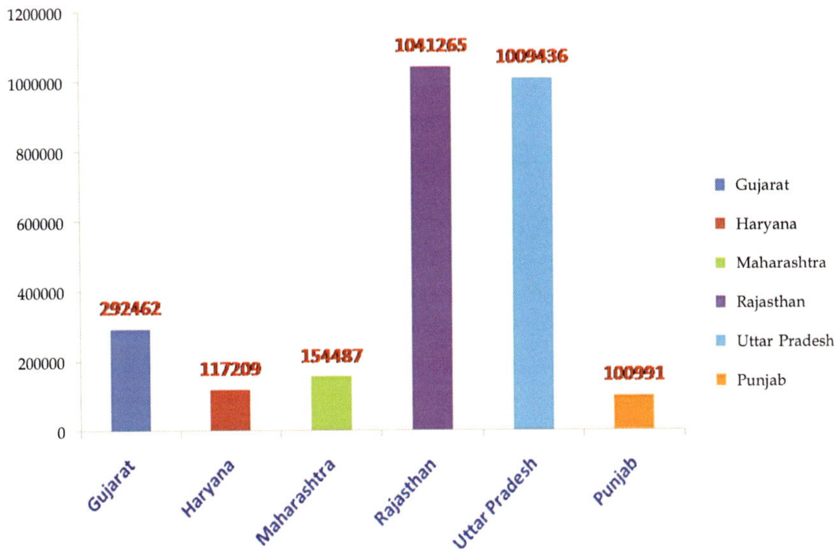

Figure 2.3 Number stray cattle in Haryana and neighbouring states.

State	No. of Stray Cattle (SC)	Area KM^2	SC to Area Ratio
Gujarat	292462	196025	1.49
Haryana	117209	44212	2.65
Maharashtra	154487	307713	0.50
Rajasthan	1041265	342239	3.04
Uttar Pradesh	1009436	243,286	4.14
Punjab	100991	50,362	2.00

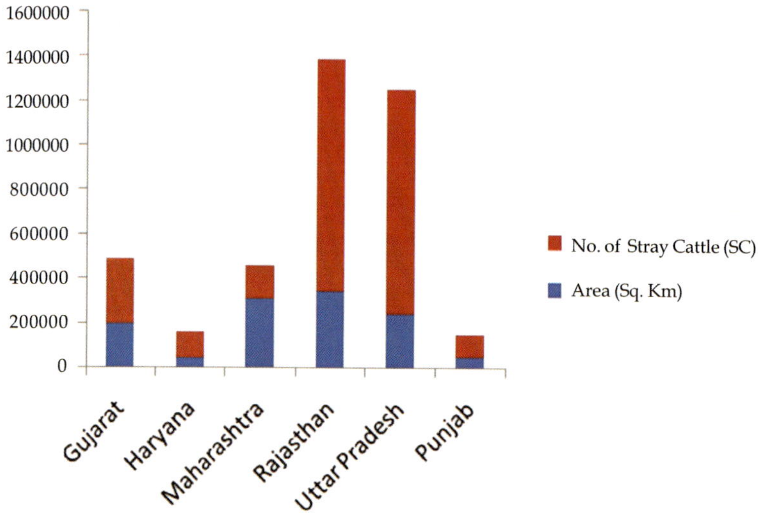

Figure 2.4 Density of stray cattle

❑❑❑

CHAPTER-3

Milk Production Trend

India ranks first in milk production, accounting for 18.5 per cent of world production, achieving an annual output of 146.3 million tones during 2014-15 as compared to 137.69 million tonnes during 2013-14 recording a growth of 6.26 per cent. Whereas, the Food and Agriculture Organization (FAO) has reported a 3.1 per cent increase in world milk production from 765 million tones in 2013 to 789 million tones in 2014. The increased production of milk has improved the per capita availability to 337 g/day but it still remains half the world average. The major concern of country is the low productivity of indigenous animals and huge dairy losses due to production related diseases in high yielding cattle.

As shown in Figure 3.1, Tamil Nadu is the largest producer of exotic/crossbred cow milk in the country with 5.82 million tonnes followed by Maharashtra with 3.72 million tonnes. Whereas, Uttar Pradesh is the largest producer of Indigenous cow milk with estimated production of 4.38 million tonnes followed by Rajasthan with 4.17 million tones. The overall productivity of indigenous cattle is very low and has been estimated as 2.50 kg/day in India.

As per BAHS, 2015 report, in Haryana there was continuous decline in number of indigenous cows in milk from 2009-10 to 2013-14 but there is trivial change in milk production (Figure 3.2). This may be due to replacement of native Hariana cows in large numbers that is dual purpose breed with famous dairy breeds like Sahiwal and Tharparker, as farmers are giving more emphasis to high producing animals. It is practically very difficult on their part to keep low producing animals for livelihood. So, this is an area of concern and a big challenge. Government/SAU/SVU/Reseach Institutes has to take a very serious initiatives to adopt our very beautiful and bold germplam (Hariana cattle) suitable to harsh agro-climatic conditions of Haryana.

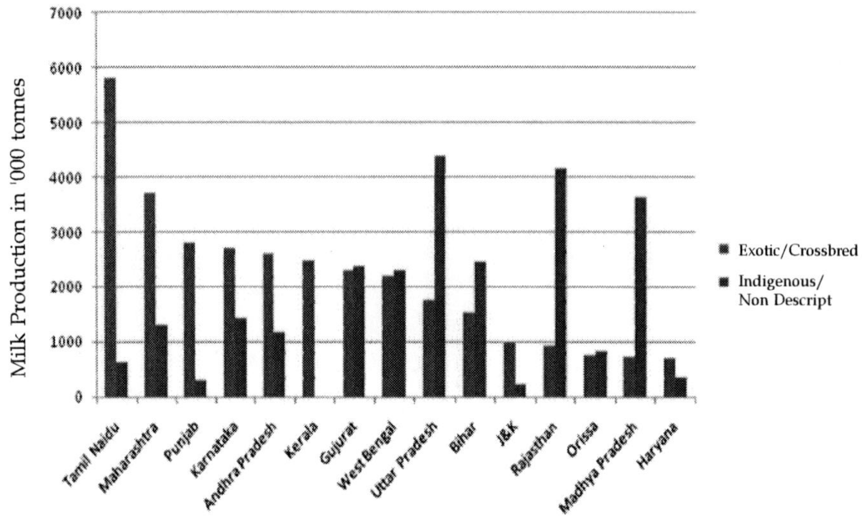

Figure 3.1 Milk production variation by indigenous and exotic/ crossbred cows in selected states for the year 2013-14

State	Exotic/ Crossbred	Indigenous/Non Descript
Tamil Naidu	5822	636
Maharashtra	3721	1295
Punjab	2816	292
Karnataka	2708	1439
Andhra Pradesh	2608	1191
Kerala	2482	3.0
Gujurat	2299	2375
West Bengal	2218	2301
Uttar Pradesh	1758	4383
Bihar	1528	2458
J&K	993	240
Rajasthan	938	4173
Orissa	758	828
Madhya Pradesh	728	3648
Haryana	696	361

(Estimate milk production in '000 tonnes, BAHS, 2015)

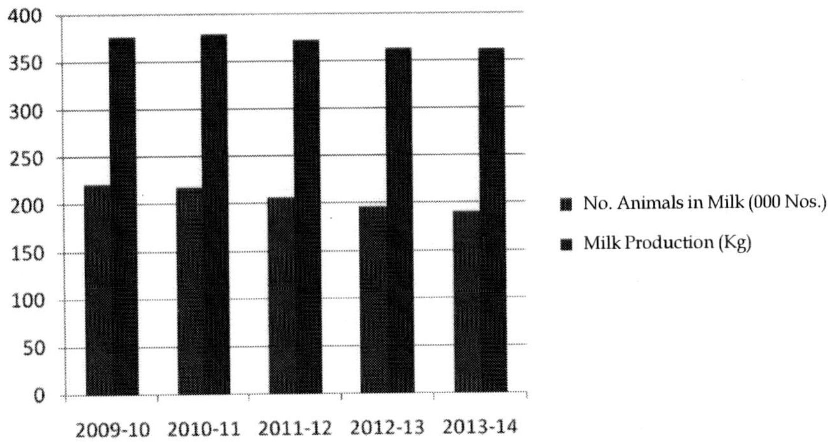

Figure 3.2 Comparative indigenous / non descript cow in milk and total milk yield statistics in Haryana (2009-10 to 2013-14)

Year	No. animals in milk (000 nos.)	Milk Production (Kg)
2009-10	220.52	376.37
2010-11	217.44	378.49
2011-12	206.57	371.29
2012-13	196.45	363.17
2013-14	189.89	361.5

The overall productivity of indigenous cattle has been estimated as 2.50 kg/day in India. In India the large number of indigenous cattle are having low productivity, which needs to be genetically improved by selective breeding. The feeding and health management are another aspects to be taken care in increasing the productivity. Though in majority of the states, Indian cattle breeds are draft in nature but a slight increase in their productivity may significantly increase the total milk production of the country as well as the livelihood of their owners.

In today's world of modernization and technologies, the utilization of cow has been raised in the field of medicine, manure, insecticide, fuel and milk. In rural areas a small number of small and marginal farmers still need the cow for agriculture and transport. They are still dependent on bullocks for their agricultural activities and rural transport though mechanization of agriculture has been noticed with varying intensity in different parts of the country.

❑❑❑

CHAPTER-4

Cattle Biodiversity of India

India is endowed with vast and varied forms of animal genetic resources that have played crucial role in augmenting agrarian economy. Traditionally, India has been a mega biodiversity center and rearing of domesticated animals. The state of world's animal genetic resources (SoW-AnGR) published by FAO in 2007 listed a total of 60 local, 8 regional transboundary and 7 international transboundary cattle breeds in India. International transboundary cattle breeds of Indian origin include Sahiwal, Gir, Red Sindhi, Ongole, Nellore and Tharparkar whereas regional transboundary breeds of Indian origin are Hariana, Kangyam, Khillari and Siri.

4.1 Breed registration

The registration process is a critical pathway for public description and documentation of genetic materials. Recognizing the need for an authentic national documentation system of valuable sovereign genetic resource with known characteristics, Indian Council of Agricultural Research (ICAR) initiated a mechanism for "Registration of Animal Germplasm" by giving temporary authority to National Bureau of Animal Genetic Resources (NBAGR), Karnal in 2007. Subsequently in 2008, ICAR constituted a Breed Registration Committee (BRC) under the chairmanship of Deputy Director General (Animal Science), ICAR. This mechanism is the sole recognized process for registration of "Animal Genetic Resources" material at national level.

As per 19th Livestock Census over 79 per cent of the cattle population is indigenous. These indigenous populations are divided into 40 recognized registered breeds by NBAGR.

Initially a total of 30 breeds were registered as extant breeds of cattle in India, subsequently ten more breeds were registered making the tally to 40. The newly registered cattle breeds included are given in Table 4.1.

Table 4.1 Newly registered cattle breeds (NBAGR)

Breed	Origin
Binjharpuri,	Odisha
Motu,	Odisha
Ghumsuri	Odisha
Khariar	Odisha
Kosali	Chhattisgarh
Malnad Gidda	Karnataka
Pullikulam	Tamil Nadu
Belahi	Haryana
Gangatiri	Uttar Pradesh and Bihar
Badri	Uttarakhand

As per the breed survey report 2013 by department of animal husbandry, dairying and fishery (DADF), total number of indigenous animals were 151.17 million out of which 113.25 million were non-descript. Number of pure indigenous animals belonging to different breeds were 17.84 million and 20.07 million were graded animals. The highest contribution is from non-descript category of animals which is 74.9 per cent of the total Indigenous cattle Out of the remaining 25.1 per cent, 4.2 per cent contribution is from Hariana Breed followed by Gir and Sahiwal contributing over 3per cent each. Besides, Kankrej breed contributed 2 per cent and other breeds such as Kosali, Khillar, Hallikar, Malvi and Bachaur also contributed over 1per cent to the total indigenous cattle.

The vulnerable breeds are Mewati, Siri, Bargur. The endangered breeds are Krishna Valley, Punganur, Vechur contributing less than 0.03 per cent of indigenous cattle (Table 4.2).

Figure 4.2 reveals that our dairy cattle breed needs immediate attention and proper breeding strategies incorporating various reproductive bio techniques for conservation and propagation.

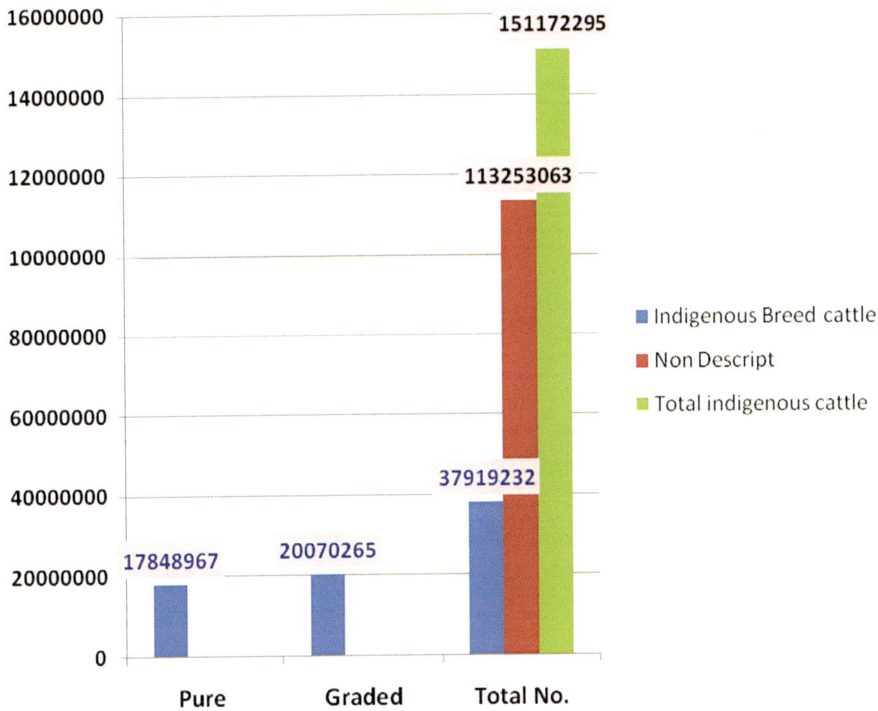

Figure 4.1 Number of animals under indigenous cattle

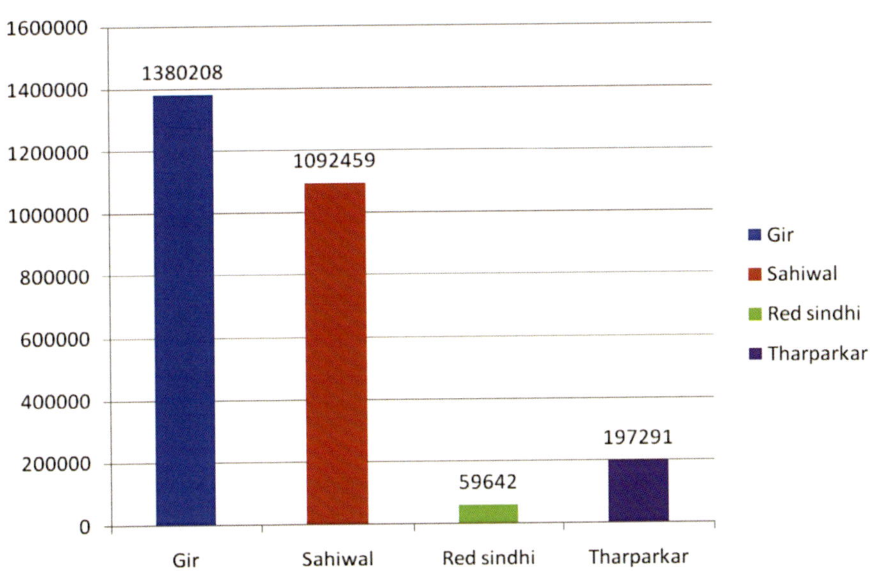

Figure 4.2 Number of pure animals of dairy cattle breeds in India

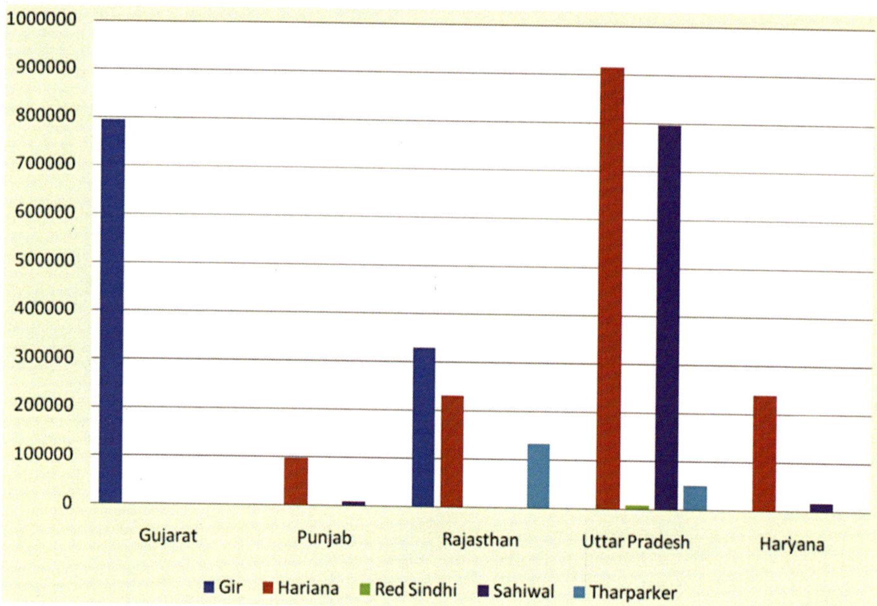

Figure 4.3 Number of animals of important breeds of cattle in Haryana and neighboring states

Breeds	Gujarat	Punjab	Rajasthan	Uttar Pradesh	Haryana
Gir	794077	108	329035	461	0
Hariana	0	96099	230582	914927	238524
Red Sindhi	0	0	0	7053	0
Sahiwal	0	8811	972	797171	17050
Tharparkar	0	906	132352	50078	697

Animals in numbers

Comparative statistics in figure 4.3 reveals that number of dairy cattle breeds in Haryana is not up to the mark. It may be due to more demand of buffalo milk and farmers are giving more emphasis to Buffalo farming. So, important dairy breeds like Sahiwal, Gir, Tharparkar needs promotion at farmers and institution level. Red Sindhi breed almost extinct and needs serious attentions, only few animals were available in Uttar Pradesh. Gir breed is gaining popularity day by day and has been adopted by various institutional, organized and commercial herds in various states.

Most of the breeds of cattle are maintained at state owned organized farms where information on growth, production and reproduction parameters is recorded and maintained. There are very few farms where performance parameters on breeds maintained are recorded regularly. Information on some of the breeds has also been collected through field surveys.

However, there are still some breeds which neither have any organized farm nor any systematic survey has been conducted. Their performance records which are essential for planning breed improvement programmes are not available.

❑❑❑

CHAPTER-5

Production Systems

Indian cattle are reared under varying production systems. In recent years, many large sized dairy farms have emerged in the country which is mainly concentrating the husbandry of crossbred/exotic cattle under high input-high output production system. This is also called as intensive or industrial production system. In this production system high milk producing animals are kept on scientific lines with stall feeding and advanced management.

Another production system which is prevailing in India is crop-livestock production system, in which few cows, bullocks and followers are kept by the farmers. In this production system the productivity of the animals is low to medium and kept on grazing with the small amount of stall feeding with crop residue and kitchen waste. Under this production system the milk is partly consumed by the farmer's family and partly sold. The indigenous breeds of dual purpose of cattle or non-descript animals are generally kept under this system. This is the targeted area that needs immediate focus and action plan to adopt these farmers for conservation and propagation of our indigenous animals, ultimately uplifting the socio-economic status of the farmers.

One more production system is also prevailing in the country which is known as pastoral system. In this system big herds of cattle are maintained and kept on migration for more than six months in a year. The migratory herds of Gir, Kankrej and Pullikulam are very common. In this system the animals migrate due to paucity of feed and fodder in their native tract. Therefore, the herds migrate in search of feed and fodder during lean months. Cattle movement is a very serious issue requiring legal framework.

❑❑❑

CHAPTER-6

Reasons of Breed Dilution / Decline

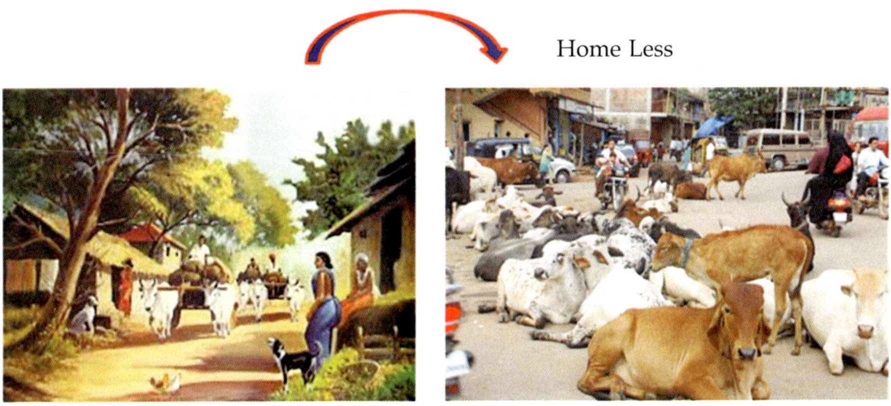

The total indigenous cattle population decreased by 8.94 per cent and crossbred population increased by 20.18 per cent compared to 18th Livestock census, (2007). The extinction rate has increased a hundredfold over the last century.

"In India the purity of the breeds is not maintained due to unplanned breeding in the villages and Gaushalas which leads to further deterioration of the Indian cow standards and thus bringing the status of cow further down".

The main reasons are as under:

a) **Cross breeding**: The efforts have been made to increase the country's milk production by introducing exotic germplasm of superior genetic merit through cross breeding. The cross breeding has been widely used as a major force for achieving rapid genetic change to increase animal productivity than selection within breeds.

b) **Mechanization**: The large scale mechanization after 1970 has reduced the requirement of draught animal power. Thus draught breeds of cattle have lost there utility and became economically unviable because of their low milk production ability.

c) **Preference to buffaloes**: Farmers are now a days preferring buffaloes over cattle because buffaloes are more viable economically.

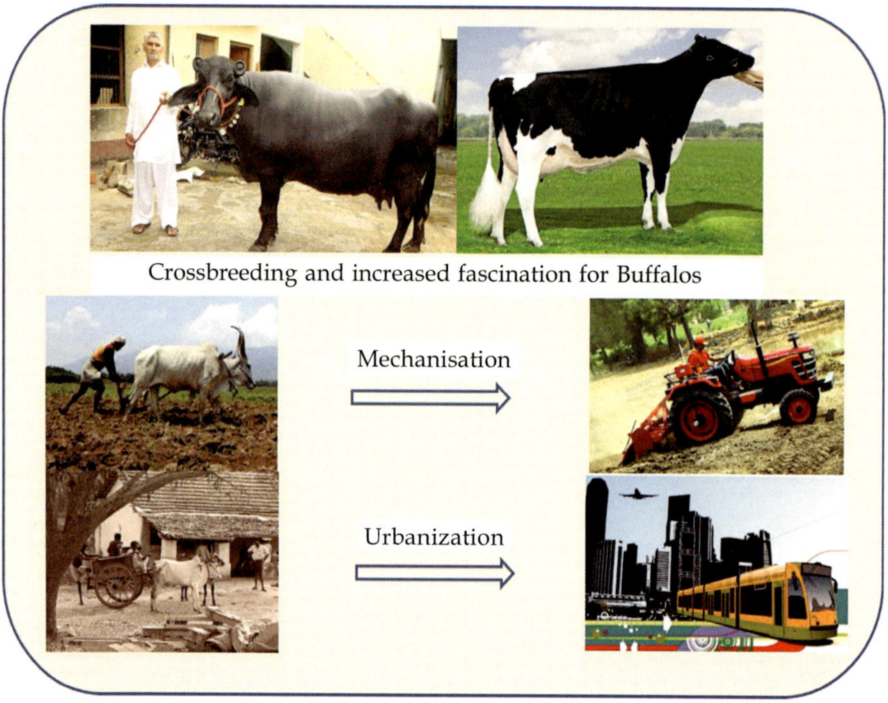

Crossbreeding and increased fascination for Buffalos

d) **Upgrading:** There had been unrestricted interbreeding among different breeds particularly in rural areas. The native breeds are crossed with superior breed for better economic returns. This has resulted into the mixture of various breeds. e.g. Tharparkar with Hariana, Sahiwal with Red Sindhi, etc.

e) **Purpose based farming system**: The different breeds of indigenous cattle serve different purposes of the owner viz milk, draught and dual. Therefore, the breeds that do not serve the purpose are neglected.

f) **Economic viability**: The economically viable breed is automatically conserved. There are certain breeds which have lost their utility due to poor performance and declining economic return to farmers. e.g.:Hariana, Mewati, Kankatha, Kherigarh, Bachur cattle.

g) **Unplanned mating:** it is happening due to lack of breeding policies and lack of knowledge on the part of farmers regarding importance of a breed.

❑❑❑

CHAPTER-7

Past / Ongoing Genetic Improvement Programmes

During the post-independence era, the Government undertook various measures towards improvement and development of the indigenous breeds in which conservation, as such, was not the area of primary concern. Broad policy frame work for cattle breeding in the country was laid down in mid-sixties, which was generally accepted and subsequently endorsed by the National Commission on Agriculture in 1976. The recommended policy envisaged improvement of indigenous breeds in their breeding tract through selective breeding and their use for upgrading the non-descript stock.

Crossbreeding was initially restricted to hilly areas and areas with preponderance of non-descript cattle. But, irresistible demand for crossbred cattle necessitated the expansion of crossbreeding programme nationwide - even in the home tracts of pure indigenous breeds. This has resulted in dilution of our valuable indigenous breeds like Ongole, Hariana, Tharparkar, Gir and Kankrej.

Castration of stray bulls and expansion of artificial insemination network were simultaneously adopted as strategic framework. The programme generally included opening of herd books for selected breeds, establishment and strengthening of breeding farms for indigenous breeds, setting up of bull centres for natural service with indigenous bulls, milk yield competitions, livestock shows, assistance to Gaushalas, etc.

In India, all types of breeding syatems are being used for genetic improvement in cattle. Selective breeding, Unstructured breeding, grading up and to certain extent crossbreeding.

7.1 Progeny-testing (PT) scheme

PT was started in the Third Five-Year Plan to ensure identification of superior Hariana bulls tested on the basis of performance of their progeny rather than only the dam's yield. In order to achieve higher genetic gain test bulls were used through artificial insemination. There are some field progeny testing programmes for indigenous breeds of cattle by the Government, Cooperatives dairies, Research Institutes and NGOs. Even these programmes are deficient for want of requisite performance recording. Most of ongoing progeny testing programmes are dependent on institutional herds, leaving out good animals possessed by the farming community. However, the number of bulls tested and selected is too few to make any appreciable impact on genetic improvement. Now question arise why so? Crores of rupee we spent, numbers of years we wasted but still we are at base level. **It is right time to fix responsibility and review critically the neglected facts.**

7.2 AICRP/Network project

Projects aimed for conservation and genetic improvement conservation of indigenous AnGR are being undertaken at specific institutes of Indian Council of Agricultural Research (ICAR) and in collaboration with the State Agricultural Universities. Such activities have also been taken up by State and Central Government Farms, NDDB and some NGOs including Gaushalas. The project is being implemented in the home tract of indigenous breeds maintained under farm and field conditions. Presently, implemented for three important breeds viz., Gir, Kankrej and Sahiwal. The project envisages establishment of germplasm (G.P.) and data recording units (D.R.) for each breed in collaboration with the State Agricultural Universities and ICAR institutes. The young bulls born out of nominated mating of elite cows at the germplasm centre are to be progeny tested using animal and farm facilities existing at the Data Recording Units/associated herds.

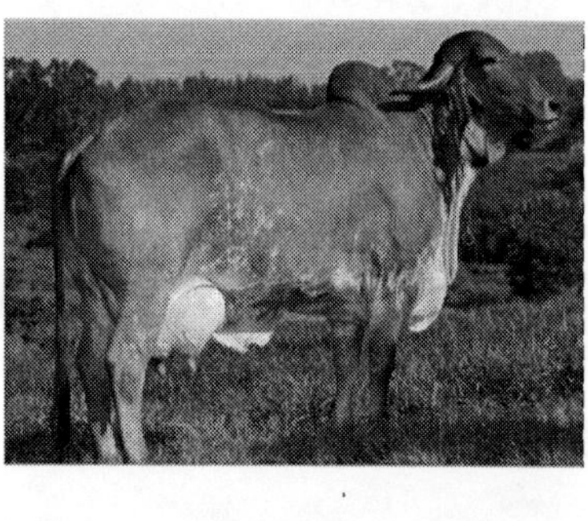

Gir: The germplam unit (GP) of Gir cattle is located at Cattle Breeding Farm, Junagadh Agricultural University, Junagadh (Gujarat) and the data recording (DR) units are located at 14 farmers herds and three organised associated herds.

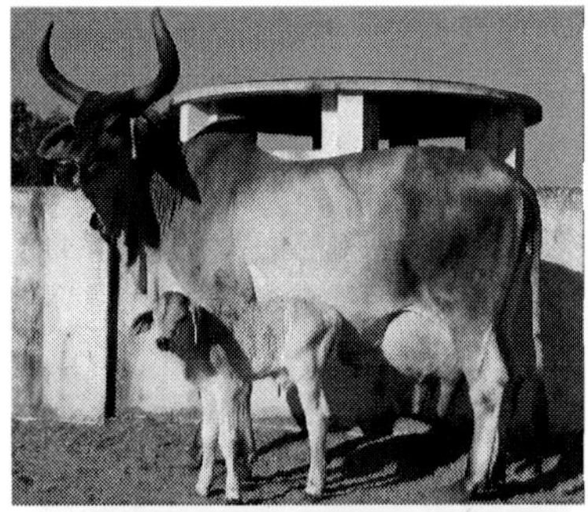

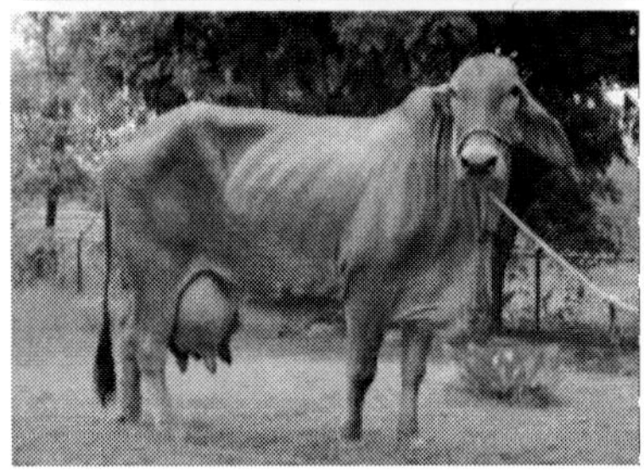

Kankrej: The GP unit of Kankrej cattle is located at Livestock Research Station, Sardarkrushinagar Dantiwada Agricultural University, Sardarkrushinagar, Gujarat and five DR units consisting of organized farms and farmers' herds have been identified under the project.

Sahiwal: The GP unit of Sahiwal breed is located at National Dairy Research Institute, Karnal and five DR units are located at :

a) Government Livestock Farm-I, Hissar

b) GADVASU, Ludhiana,

c) Shri Gaushala Trust, Bhiwani,

d) G.B. Pant University of Agriculture and Technology, Pantnagar,

e) Cattle Breeding Farm, Anjora, Durg, Chhattisgarh.

7.3 Herd registration programme

The primary aim is to identify elite germplasm for further improvement in milk production. Indigenous cattle breeds covered are Gir, Kankrej, Hariana and Ongole. Under the scheme incentives for rearing of elite cows and their male calves is given to the owners of the elite animals.

7.4 Intensive cattle development project

Intensive Cattle Development Project (ICDP), was started in 1966-67. It was envisaged to cover 0.1 million cows and take care of all aspects of development such as, breeding, feeding, disease control and extension activities.The main impact of the ICDP is genetic improvement through AI using the semen of genetically superior males.

7.5 National project for cattle and buffalo breeding (NPCBB)

The government of India initiated action in the beginning of 9th Plan in consultation with State governments and other concerned agencies with an aim to consolidate the gains achieved till VIII Plan period, to maximize returns on investments, and to ensure sustainability of operations as well as quality in breeding inputs and services. The objectives of the project include establishment of appropriate institutional structures to channel and supply high quality breeding inputs and services; setting up national standards for bulls, semen laboratories and AI services.

□□□

CHAPTER-8

Government Initiatives

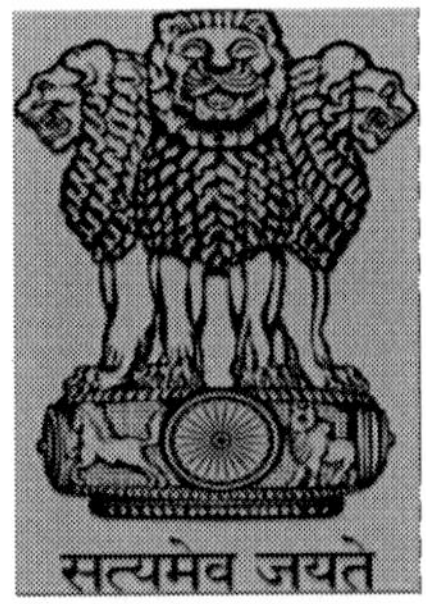

The *desi* mission of the NDA government has reached *'gaushalas'*, as the government has allotted a massive sum of **Rs 500 crore to raise strictly *'desi'* cows**. The Union Government has also launched Rashtriya Gokul Mission under the same programme for conservation and development of indigenous breeds in a focused and scientific manner.

8.1 Rashtriya gokul mission

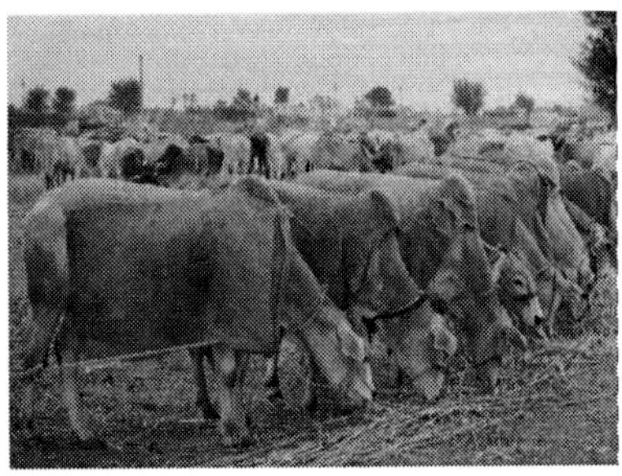

India, though being the largest producer of milk is known for the quantity of cows rather than the high yield and quality of them. Thus, the project, named 'Rashtriya Gokul Mission', aims to promote locally bred cows as they are better suited for the Indian climate and are even heat resistant. Thus, by switching to purely locally bred cows over cross-bred, it aims to increase the output of milk.

This scheme aims to even maintain the cows after they have passed their milk producing stage. Even the cow dung and cow urine will be utilised. It will be promoted as organic manure and for other purposes, such as for biogas to produce electricity.

In order to make the farmers motivated towards the new scheme, those that maintain the best cow centres will be awarded "Gopal Ratna" awards. Each cow will be given a unique identity number and all the records will be maintained in a national database.

The 'Gopal Sanghs' or the breeding facilities will aim to even escalate into a public-private partnership.

The Centre also runs a major programme for genetic upgradation called the National project for cattle and buffalo breeding.

Currently, India is falling behind the United States and New Zealand, as our output is just one-fifth compared to the two countries. The United Nations Food and Agriculture Organisation highlights that intrinsically low genetic potential and poor quality of animal nutrition are the leading problems. Thus the new scheme aims to solve these problems.

8.2 National programme for bovine breeding and dairy development (NPBBDD)

National Programme for Bovine Breeding and Dairy Development (NPBBDD) was launched by the union government in February 2014 after merging four erstwhile schemes viz., National project for cattle and buffalo breeding (NPCBB), Intensive dairy development programme (IDDP), Strengthening infrastructure for quality and clean milk production (SIQ and CMP) and assistance to cooperatives.

The Scheme had two components:

a) National Programme for Bovine Breeding (NPBB)

b) National Programme for Dairy Development (NPDD).

NPBB will focus amongst other things on extension of the Field Artificial Insemination (Al) Net work, monitoring of Al programme, development and conservation of indigenous breeds and establishment of breeders' associations and societies to encourage conservation and development of recognized indigenous breeds.

The NPDD component of NPBBDO scheme has been designed to develop infrastructure from the grass root level by providing financial and technical assistance for dairy development. NPDD will focus on creating infrastructure related to production, procurement, processing and marketing by milk unions/federations and also extension activities including training of farmers.

8.3 Gauvansh sanrakshan and Gau samvardhan' bill, 2015 (Haryana)

The bill banning the sale of beef in Haryana was passed on March 14th 2015. This Bill places a complete ban on cow slaughter in the state and also envisages the establishment of institutions to take care of stray, non-productive, infirm or injured cows. Government also aims to provide financial as well as technical support to these institutions. Through this act, the government will also promote the projects and programmes for cow conservation and protection.

❑❑❑

CHAPTER-9

Need for Conservation

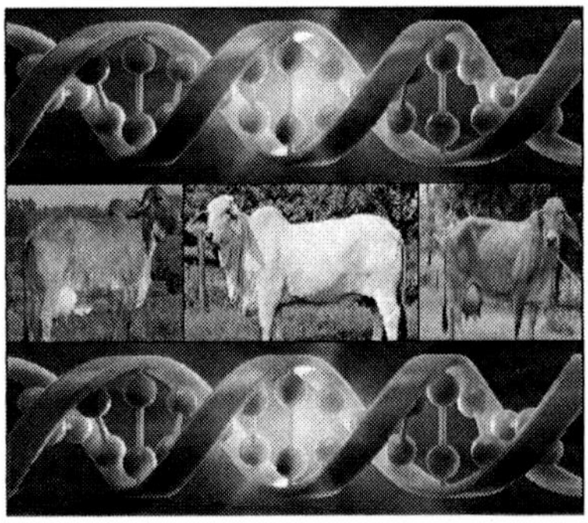

a) **Genetic insurance:** Native breeds have been developed over thousands of years and have better adaptability to harsh climate, are resistant to diseases, heat tolerant and can utilize locally available poor quality roughages. So they have unique genes or gene combinations which are associated with adaptability and producing ability under harsh environment. Thus loss of such breeds means loss of DNA sequences responsible for adaptive traits.

b) **Scientific study:** *"As somewhere something incredible waiting to be known"*. The conservation of native breeds provides useful materials in genetics, biochemistry, physiology, morphology and anatomy. It is also useful to understand the process of evolution, domestication and the effects of natural and artificial selection.

c) **Environmental considerations:** Every organism has its own role to play within an ecosystem and the loss of germplasm has adverse effect on the ecosystem which is hazardous to existence of mankind.

d) **Cultural and ethical requirements:** If a breed is not economically viable, it should be preserved for cultural and public interest of historical importance since the animal genetic resources are part of the natural heritage, culture and ecosystem. From vedic reference, cow is abode of Gods. She is Kamdhenu (desire fulfiller) personified. All the demigods reside in the body of a cow. She is receiver of the auspicious rays from all heavenly constellations. Thus it contains influences of all constellations. Wherever there is a cow, there is influence of all heavenly constellations; blessings of all Gods are there. Cow is the only divine living being that has a surya ketu nadi (vein connected to sun) passing through her backbone. Therefore the cow's milk, butter and ghee have golden hue. These salts are present in the cow milk and cow's other body fluids, which miraculously cures many diseases

e) **Energy source:** India has a number of good draught breeds of cattle used to perform a number of agricultural operations before intensification of mechanized agriculture. However, a non-renewable source of energy may be exhausted sooner or later. In such situation animal draught power will be required and hence these breeds should not be allowed to become extinct.

9.1 Superiority of desi cow and its products

Milk Ghee Curd	A2
Dung	Organic Farming
	Dried Dung Cakes
	Thermal Insulation in Cold Weather
	Shields Radiation and Repels Insects
	Biogas
	Good Disinfectant
Urine	Pesticide, Medicinal Properties

According to the Animal Laws in India, cows cannot be slaughtered. Practically slaughtering of cows is slaughtering the economy of the country. The key for village economy of India is Indigenous cattle and can provide immediate solutions to stressed agriculture farming. Cows and bulls are used in fields and their dung and urine are used to make compost, medicine and other health products. Applications and utilities of cow products are as follows.

9.1.1 *Animal draught power*

In India draught power is utilized mainly in agriculture for ploughing and threshing. The bullock carts are used for carrying the loads for agricultural purposes as well as also contribute in transport of rural people from one place to another. Bullocks are playing a

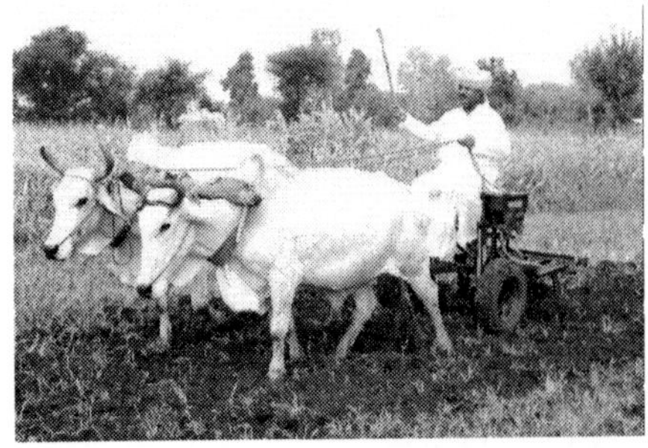

significant role in agricultural production of India as even today more than 60 per cent of agriculture is dependent on bullock power. In India more than 80 per cent of cattle breeds have been evolved for draft purposes. The Hariana and Nagori in North, Khillar in West, Hallikar, Kangyam, Amritmahal and Umblacherry in South are the famous draft breeds of India. Bullocks are generally used for draft purposes, however, in south and northeast states dry cows are also used for draft purposes. Many researchers reported that 0.70 horse power per day is generated from a good breed bullock whereas, 0.40 horse power from non-descript bullock and bullocks are fully utilized for 100 days in a year. Therefore, 1575 crores kilo watt hour energy is generated from the bullocks. The tractor has the utility for the farmers having land holding of 4 hectares or more but in India 75 per cent farmers are having the land holding less than 2 hectares, thereby the bullock power is the basis of their agricultural livelihood. This is the reason that more than 60 per cent of Indian agricultural operations are dependent on the bullock power.

Keeping in view the geographical diversity, purchasing power and land holding of Indian farmers it would be rightly stated that in the coming years the utility of bullock power will continue in India.

9.1.2 *Ayurveda*

In addition to the above uses, cattle in India are valued for the production of Panchgavya prepared from its products and byproducts. Panchgavya means five elements i.e. Milk, ghee, curd, urine, dung. It is claimed that the medicines which are made up of panchgavya are free from the harmful chemicals.

Panchagavya is the most important medicinal combination used in ayurvedic medicine. As per Ayurvedic classics, it is good for health. Panchagavya Ayurved Chikitsa for human beings is gaining importance. It also has other valuable medicinal implications for cure of Asthma, skin diseases, weakness, allergy, diabetes, etc.

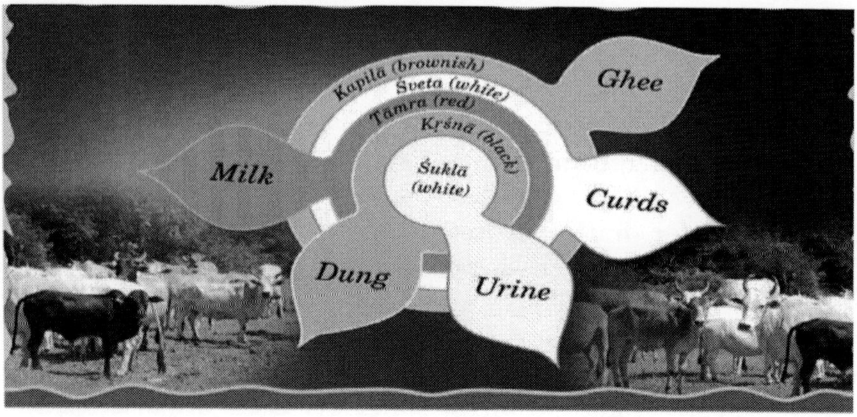

Panchagvya Ayurved Chikitsa for veterinary applications needs research support. The Kamdhenu ark is reported to be used in treatment of renal failure of animals. Curd helping in controlling cholesterol, it is helpful in treatment of cancer. As per Ayurvedic classics, it is useful in various kinds of systemic, physical & mental disorders. It helps in sustaining the age for long time & maintains body biochemistry in its optimum level.

9.1.3 *Indigenous cattle milk*

Cow milk mentioned as best milk among all. As per Ayurvedic classics, cow milk is useful in various diseases. Further, it increases vital energy & immune power of the person. Chemical Composition wise, it is having fat, carbohydrate and minerals. The nutritional value of milk of Indian cows (if not fed with grass polluted with chemical fertilizer and plastic) on the other hand is the highest along with many curative properties against many diseases.

Finding of life sciences has proved that milk of Indian cows contain an amino acid **Proline** which is strongly bonded to another amino acid **Insoleucine**. Such milk, called as A2 milk has the capability to fight against diseases and disorders of human body like obesity, joint pain, asthma, mental problems, etc. A2 milk contains high levels of Omega 3 that cleans the cholesterol deposits of blood vessels.

A2 vs A1 Milk: Indian survey

Beta-casein is the most polymorphic bovine milk protein gene with 13 known protein variants (Roginski, 2003). The most common forms of beta-casein in dairy cattle breeds are A1 and A2, while B is less common, and A3 and C are rare (Farrell *et al.*, 2004). Polymorphism at codon 67 of the beta-casein gene: CCT!CAT causes a substitution of amino acid proline (A2) by histidine (A1). This difference in amino acid sequence might generate conformational changes in the secondary protein structure and therefore affect physical properties of casein micelles. The presence of histidine residue at codon 67 makes A1 and B variants exclusively vulnerable to gastrointestinal proteolysis digestion to release bioactive peptide, betacasomorphin-7 (BCM-7) (Cieslinska *et al.*, 2007; De Noni 2008). Bovine BCM-7 has been implicated in potential risk of human ischemic heart diseases (McLachlan, 2001; Laugesen and Elliott, 2003), insulin-dependent diabetes (Elliott *et al.*, 1999; Laugesen and Elliott, 2003) atherosclerosis (Tailford *et al.*, 2003) and sudden infant death syndrome (Sun et al. 2003). No such survey has been carried out in India so far. No doubt all these are multi-factorial diseases but we made an effort to correlate the effect of A1 milk in India (Table 9.1). Surprisingly, people from states where there is more contribution of milk from crossbreds, have high incidence of diabetes and hypertension.

Table 9.1 Indian Survey

STATE	Per cent Diabetes Suspected	Per cent Hypertension Suspected	CB	ND	Buffalo	Goat
			Per cent Milk contribution			
Sikkim	13.67	18.16	80	20	0.3	-
Madhya Pradesh	2.57	2.87	7	38	49	6
Haryana	4.8	6.24	9	5	85	1
Punjab	9.36	9.26	28	3.3	68	.7
J&K	5.61	8.21	61	15	18	6
Karnataka	9.36	3.57	44	25	30	1
West Bengal	6.55	3.22	44	48	5	3

(NPCDCS, 2013 & BAHS, 2014)

9.1.4 *Urine*

Drinking cow urine, (Gaumutra) on a regular basis (and prescribed quantity) helps the human body fight hundreds of diseases and increase immunity. India's oldest holy texts including the Vedas have considered cows as a mobile dispensary and Gau Mutra as a medicine

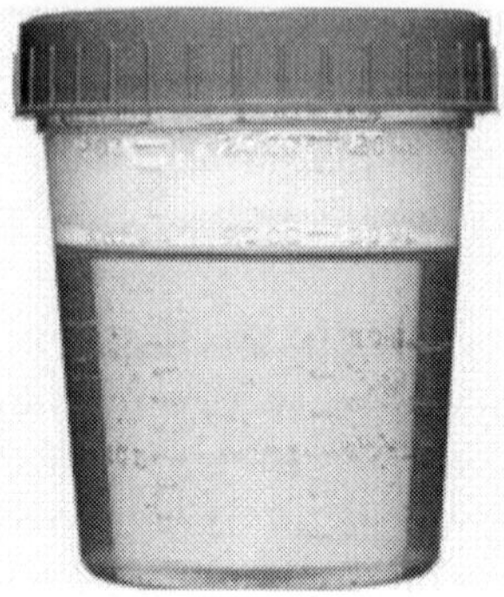

to cure even the incurable diseases. The Cow Urine Treatment and Research Center, Indore has conducted a lot of research in the past few years and reached the conclusion that it is capable of curing diabetes, blood pressure, asthma, psoriasis, eczema, heart attack, blockage in arteries, fits, cancer, aids, piles, prostrate, arthritis, migraine, thyroid, ulcer, acidity, constipation, gynecological problems, ear and nose problems, abortion and several other diseases.

The bio-enhancer antibiotic, antifungal and antibacterial property (US patent no. 6410059), anti-allergic properties along with anti-infective and anticancer (US patent no. 6896907 and 27235262), antioxidant property (US patent no. 7718360) of cow urine has been established by Go-Vigyan Anusandhan Kendra, Nagpur. *There are many other studies on the panchgavya and cow urine distillate which clearly indicate that the properties of cow urine can be exploited for increasing the profitability of the cow owners.*

9.1.5 *Manure and fuel*

Cow dung is referred as Gomay and is considered equally holy as Gomutra and it is used to purify environment. Cow dung have anti-radiation property. Various internal and external medicinal use of cow dung is seen in classics. Cow dung is used for the production of gobar gas, methane gas, fertilizer and manure. Gobar gas produced from cow dung is eco-friendly and do not cause pollution. When the solid CO_2 is removed from gobar gas, the methane gas is obtained. This methane gas can be used for driving the automobiles and vehicles. Cow dung can be used as manure and by using organic manure prepared from cow dung, we may get freedom from the harmful and side effects which are caused by the use of chemical based fertilizers as well as control the insects and pests which may damage the crop.

9.1.6 *Organic farming*

Organic farming system in India is not new and is being followed from ancient time. It is a method of farming system which primarily aimed at cultivating the land and raising crops in such a way, as to

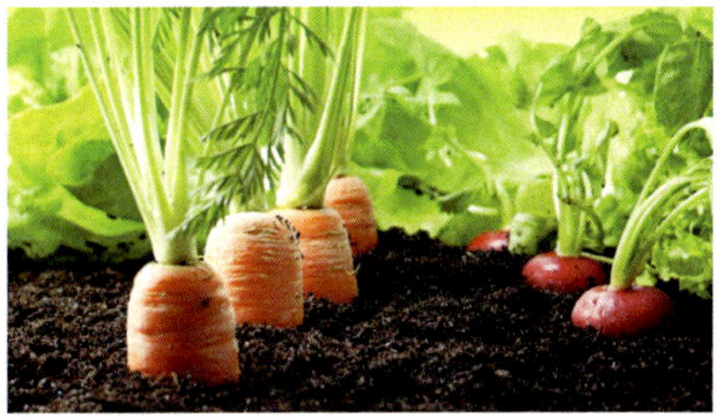

keep the soil alive and in good health by use of organic wastes (crop, animal and farm wastes, aquatic wastes) and other biological materials along with beneficial microbes (biofertilizers) to release nutrients to crops for increased sustainable production in an eco friendly pollution free environment.

The concept of organic agriculture has been perceived differently by the farmers of the developing and of the least developed countries. To most of the farmers in countries like India it implies the use of organic manures and natural methods of plant protection instead of synthetic fertilizers and plant protection chemicals.

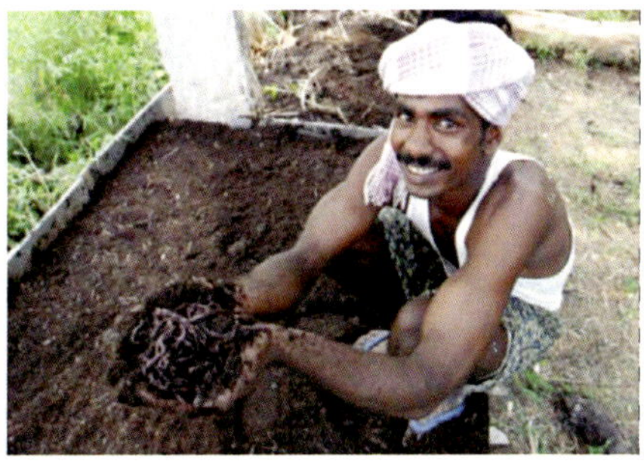

From vedic period it is believed that "Gomaye Vaste Lakshmi" It means Goddess of wealth resides in Cow Dung. It is true also because enormous wealth can be obtained from cow dung by its proper utilization. The preparations like vermi compost, kitniyantrak and amritpani from cowdung and cow urine. The large number of farmers are using above products. The experiences show that by using these products, the land has become more fertile which resulted in increase of production. Moreover, costwise also, it is economical than the chemical fertilizers/ Insecticide. The gobar gas product and its use as energy source along with farm fertilizer application is well known.

❑❑❑

CHAPTER-10

Action Plan for Sustainable Conservation and Utilization of Indigenous Cattle

Many local cattle breeds continue to represent the livelihood of rural populations. They fulfill a much wider range of functions and provide a large number of products. Their maintenance is ecologically more sustainable, especially in marginal environments. Indigenous animals are being maintained by farmers in small herds. The number of holding for all the breeds is very large. They are well adapted to the local conditions under low input system and are providing employment and livelihood to a large section of the society under the rural conditions. The diversity of our valuable germplasm helps them to produce under diverse environment. commercialization of animal husbandry practices is still slow in most parts of India.

10.1 National level priorities for capacity building to improve understanding of cattle genetic resources

At present, priority is being given to characterization and evaluation of indigenous cattle breeds. Surveys are being conducted in the breeding tracts through a network approach by involving various agencies. Conservation of various breeds both in-situ and ex-situ has also been taken up. Programmes for the genetic improvement of breeds are being undertaken.

Priorities areas for further improving the understanding of cattle genetic resources are:

i) Online database of indigenous cattle breeds

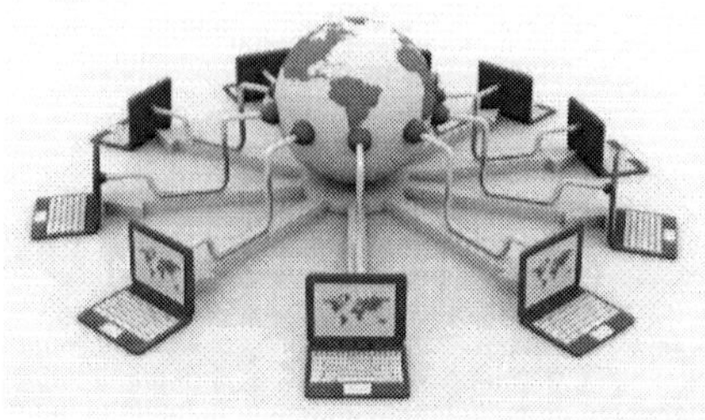

Systematic identification and data recording of all the animals at the field level is must for successful implementation of any breeding programme. In case of indigenous cattle, there is no adequate and efficient data base management system in India. This is one of the major hindrance for the genetic improvement of our cattle. So, development of a centralized online database management system is very much essential now days. This database management system should have to keep an option for farmers themselves to make the recording of their animals either through mobile applications or SMS services.

Indigenous Cattle Card (ICC)- Breed wise unique identification number must be given to all indigenous cattle, to overcome problems like indiscriminate breeding, breed dilution and unauthentic data.

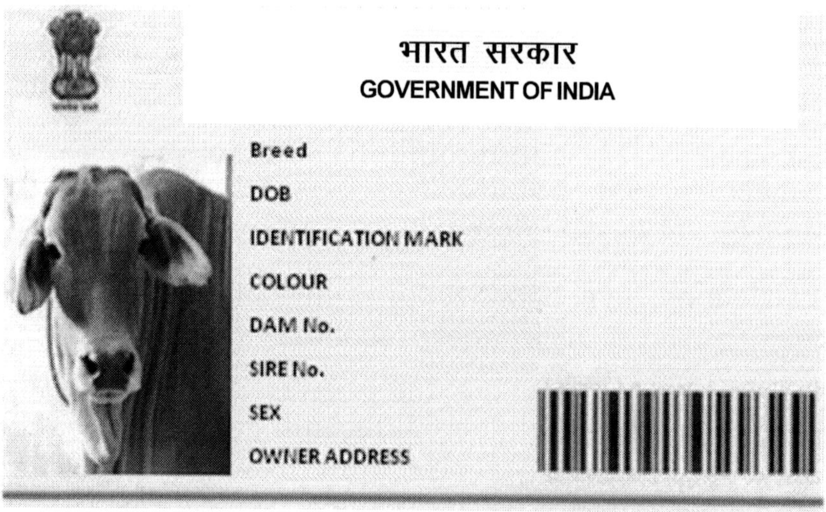

I C C - Indgenous Cattle Card (Sample)

ii) Breeding policy

Cross-breeding with exotic breeds should be totally banned in the breeding tracts of the important cattle breeds. Selective breeding and grading up must be followed strictly for indigenous cattle. Identify, the geographical boundaries of the areas where non-descript cattle should be upgraded by crossing with bulls of indigenous breeds. Once such areas are earmarked, no cross-breeding of non-descript cattle, other than with bulls of indigenous breeds, should be permitted. This measure will provide an incentive to the farmers in the breeding tracts to rear male stock of indigenous breeds up to the breeding age, as the demand will create a market for the bull semen or natural service. Consequently, the practice of disposing off the male calves will be curbed to some extent.

iii) Breed adoption

Breeds, which no longer find favour with the farmers and are near to extinction, whatever the reason may be, should be identified and these breeds should be preserved only in the institutional farms, with improved conservation technologies.

iv) Intrabull

There should be a single genetic improvement programme for each important breed at national level involving animals of farmers. Breeds, which are economically viable and are accepted by the common farmers, should be conserved through In-situ conservation using ONBS with MOET model involving large population throughout the breeding tract.

v) Community-based management of cattle genetic resources

'Putting the last first' – research driven by needs and wishes of farmers. Involvement of local communities and institutions in the design, implementation and ownership of breeding strategies.

vi) Breed parks- Initiatives must be taken to establish indigenous cattle breed parks in different states. Breed parks serve as

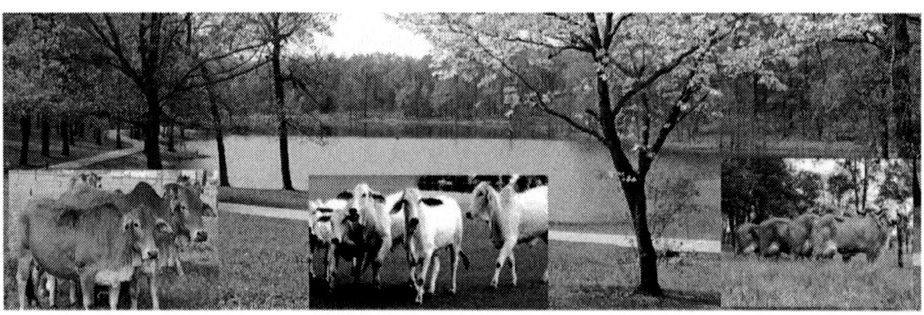

- **Education center**: Live display of different indigenous cattle will be very helpul for students, farmers and researches to learn breed differences and study animal behavior.
- **Tourist place:** Definitely attract foreign tourist, young generation and urban population to visit cattle centuries for photography, picnic, amusement, film shootings and explore their knowledge.
- **Breed Hub:** The main purpose is to conserve and propagate our valuable cattle breeds. So the chain of breed parks in India will definitely serve the purpose.

vii) Semen banks of indigenous bulls

The supply of semen of the pure indigenous cattle breed is essentially required to maintain the purity of the breed as well as genetic improvement. So, government certified semen banks of indigenous cattle and various sub units must be established so that it should be easily available at farmers door step.

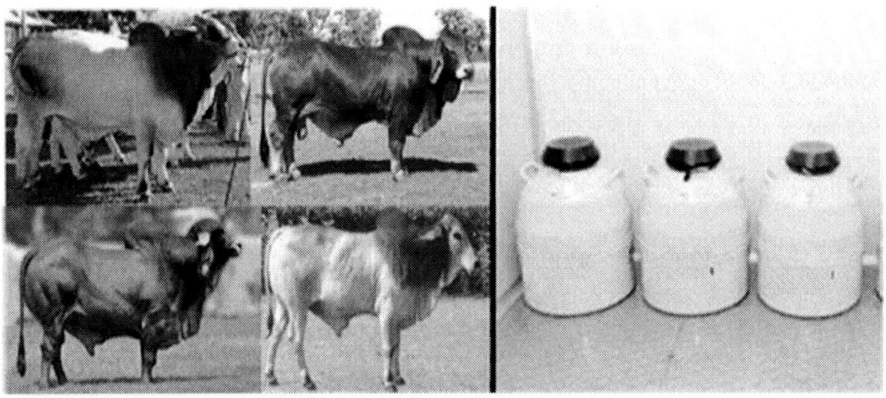

10.2 Farmers herd involvement

The best way to conserve the resources is within their native habitat *(in situ)* through active participation of livestock owners and stakeholders. The indigenous breeds especially those which are less productive can only be maintained as long as their minimum feed/ fodder requirement are met under zero or low input system specifically through grazing. It would be very important to maintain the grasslands and other feed/fodder resources, optimally under such production system. Traditionally, all the livestock were grazed on common grasslands, which were earmarked for the animals of each village. It was the responsibility of village *Panchayat* to maintain these grazing lands through controlled grazing and re-seeding and plantation to sustain the livestock. Besides this, the traditional agricultural crops were providing enough crop residues and byproducts for supplementary feeding. Livestock breeders of the arid and semi-arid regions normally take their herds to other areas during lean periods. Some of the forest areas were also utilized by the animal keepers, which has been banned for grazing in recent past for various forest development programmes. This is adversely affecting some of the breeds kept under zero input system. If grazing on one part of the forest land is allowed and at the same time on other part is banned for grazing to accomplish the development activities in the forest on rotational basis, the rearing of livestock and forest development programmes may go simultaneously.

In India, such issues can be resolved through inter-departmental negotiations at national as well as state levels.

10.2.1 *Purity of breeds*

The supply of breeding males/semen of breeds are essentially required to maintain the purity of the breed as well as genetic improvement. Farmers should be trained to develop the male progenies born to elite females of the breed for breeding purposes. The farmers should be made aware of the uniqueness of the breed and importance of maintaining purity of the breeds. Through breed shows/ competitions, the owners of good animals of the breed must be honoured at regular intervals.

10.2.2 *Incentives to farmers*

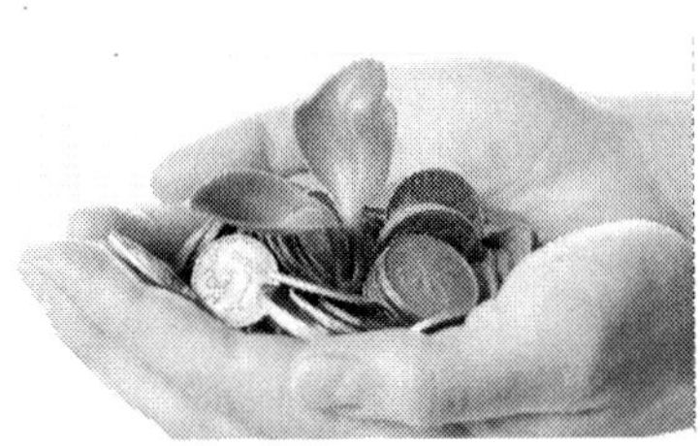

The breeds which are on the verge of extinction can be preserved by offering suitable incentives to the farmers who own such breed animals. The objective is to compensate the animal keepers for the difference in levels of production between the breed under consideration and the replacement breed under the same animal management system and agro-ecosystem. This will attract the farmers and will ensure the conservation of the breed.

However, the incentives are subject to the political decisions and are unlikely to be sustained for long term.

10.2.3 *Understanding market, dynamics*

a) Center for dung and urine collection

There is an urgent need to establish dung and urine collection centres at various places linked to ayurhubs (Patanjali, Dabur etc). Services must be provided at farmers door step i.e daily collection of dung and urine at set price for encouraging farmers to keep even non-lactating animals.

b) A2 + Organic Milk

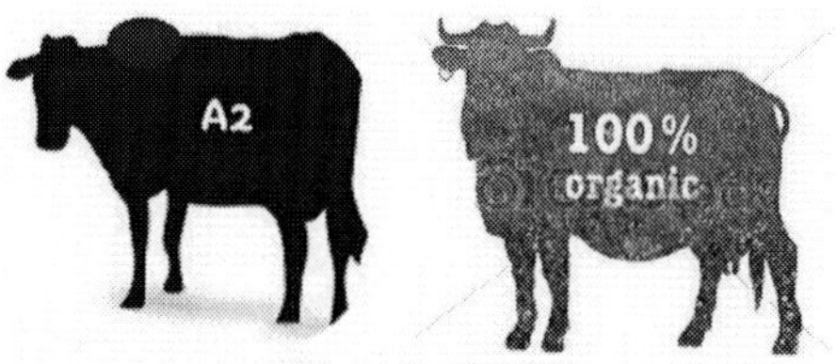

In field conditions, indiscriminate use of antibiotic on animals leads to serious consequences as antibiotics residues coming in milk leading serious health issues. Our indigenous animals are resistant to many diseases. Irrespective of A2 milk, supply of organic milk after validation will increase market value and demand.

c) Marketing facilities of breeds

Many progressive/commercial dairy farmers are interested in different indigenous breeds (e.g. Sahiwal) for commercial milk production, but they are unable to fixed the whereabouts of sale/ purchase of these breeds. Further, as pure breeds are only maintained at Govt./Institutional farms which are not capable of supplying the required animals for a dairy. Such limitations posses hinderence in adoption of superior indigenous dairy breeds like Sahiwal in commercial farms. Therefore, a national platform/website must be made accessible to all farmers/extension scientists, where livestock owners can sell or purchase required of various breeds animals. These websites must be like commercial websites used for selling and purchasing of different households like Quickrr, OLX, etc.

d) Indigenous cattle information center/ Mobile application

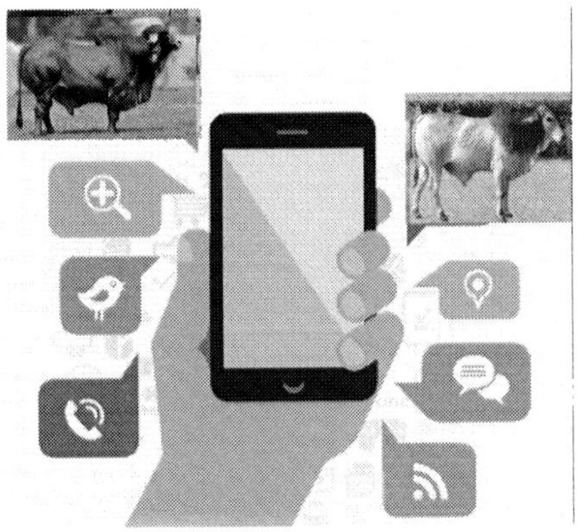

An Counselling cum Call centre/information centre/ Mobile App. should be established on indigenous breeds of cattle and it should have all the information about their distribution, farming practices, physical and molecular characteristics of the breeds, information of breed's herds and availability of elite breeding male and female cattle etc. The information also needs to be updated periodically and easily available to all.

10.3 *In situ* conservation model involving institutional herds

In situ conservation of farm animal breeds by establishing breed specific farms involves huge investment on infrastructure and resources. Due to limited facilities and budget constraints, such *in situ* conservation programs are limited to a small population.

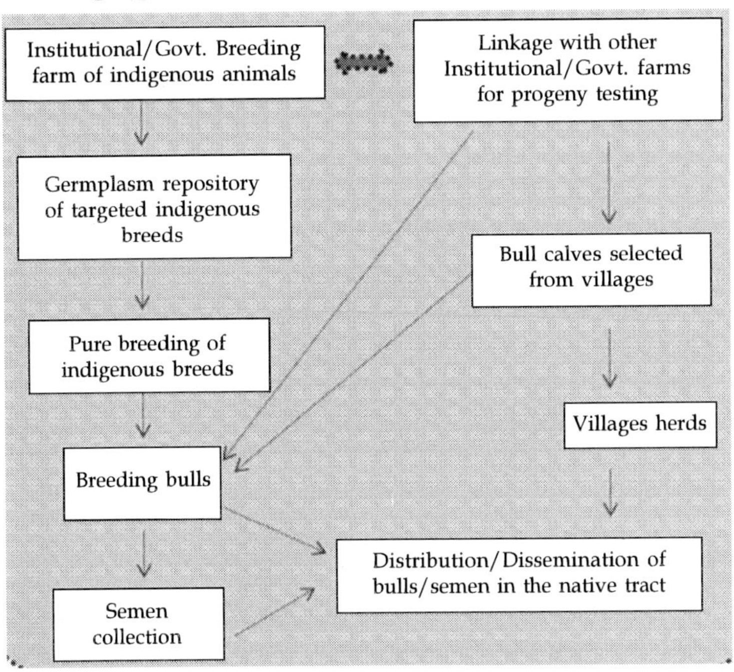

Figure 10.1 *In situ* conservation model involving institutional herds

The animals should be identified from the institutional herd and farmers' households, particularly females on the basis of true to breed characteristics and performance traits (for milk production, draft power and adaptation) and tagged.

Regular performance recording shall be followed. In addition to females, bulls (preferably at least 1 per 10 to 20 females) should be identified and tagged. The owners of candidate bulls may be provided an incentive per female per year for rearing the animals and retaining purebred animals. The selected females should be mated/inseminated with a bull/semen of the same breed. The farmers rearing the male progeny born from these pure bred females up to six months should be given extra incentives.

A total of at least 40 unrelated young males would be selected (>50 males are preferred). If AI technology is available, the selected young males shall be purchased by the development agency, for rearing males until maturity, and then training them for semen production. At maturity a total of 25 males (depending on the size of the female population) are selected on the basis of growth, semen quality and freezability. A minimum of 2000 semen doses from each male may be collected, cryopreserved and used for breed improvement and conservation. The surplus breeding males are distributed to the farmers for natural mating in the breeding tract.

The existing farms of indigenous breeds should be declared as germplasm repositories and used for production of quality bulls/sires and semen. Efforts should be made to establish one such farm for each breed in the native breed tract.

Only pure breeding of the indigenous breeds should be practiced at these farms. Facilities for frozen semen production should be developed in such farms so as to disseminate the germplasm from pure breeding bulls typical to the breed in the native tract. Associated herd progeny testing program may also be initiated if there are more such farms available for an indigenous breed so as to couple the conservation program with systematic genetic improvement.

10.4 Gaushala conservation model

There are over 4000 gaushalas in the country maintaining animals of different indigenous breeds. At present, Rajasthan, Haryana, Gujarat, Bihar and Punjab have 678, 408, 231, 148 and 167 gaushalas, respectively. However, they do not have sufficient resources and technical back up in conserving and improving these animals.

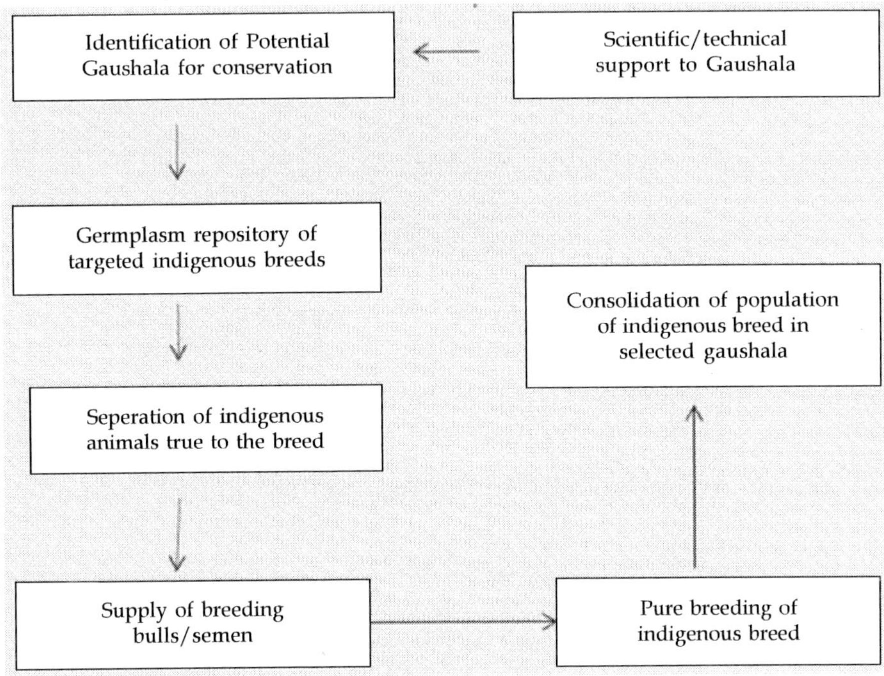

Figure 10.2 *In situ* conservation model involving Gaushalas

The strategy should be to use these gaushalas in consolidating and increasing the population of purebred animals of specific indigenous breeds. Gaushalas with potential to participate in conservation programs should be identified and supported technically and financially to maintain these indigenous breeds. An agreement and regular check should be made with the participating gaushalas not revert to crossbreeding or other such practices which may dilute the breed. Gaushalas should be advised to segregate the animals true to the indigenous breed to be conserved and breed them with semen of the same breed. Either purebred breeding bulls or frozen semen from bull stations and other necessary supplement inputs should be given to these gaushalas free of cost. Also, gaushalas may be encouraged in identifying certain products of the indigenous breeds so as to increase their economic value. Scientific and technical support may be given to the gaushalas in identifying the peculiarity of such products from indigenous animal breeds.

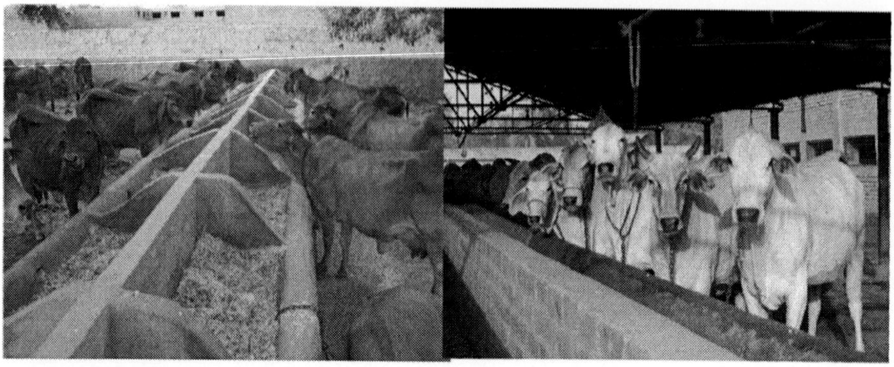

The following actions could be strictly undertaken to utilize these progressive Gaushalas:

a) Identification of the Gaushalas with a large number of purebred animals for breeds at risk.

b) Financial support to the Gaushalas shall be ensured to develop infrastructure necessary to transform these Gaushalas from rehabilitation centres into genetic resource centres.

c) The animal within each Gaushala has to be grouped and house separately the purebred and non-purebred animals.

d) Implementation of **online data base management system** for identification, performance recording and breeding programmes for the selected animals.

e) Improvement of the purebred stock has to be through selective breeding. The excess purebred stock shall be distributed to the local community targeting farmers that are willing to continue pure breeding of the animals.

10.5 Conservation model involving farmers

The conservation of indigenous cattle under sustainable management at the farmers household is one of the most effective and practical way of conserving the animals with minimum of inputs. This approach also does not involve large economic inputs and would be feasible under field conditions. However, as there has been change in the management and production system after intensification and mechanization of agriculture, major emphasis should be on the economics of the livestock breed that needs to be conserved.

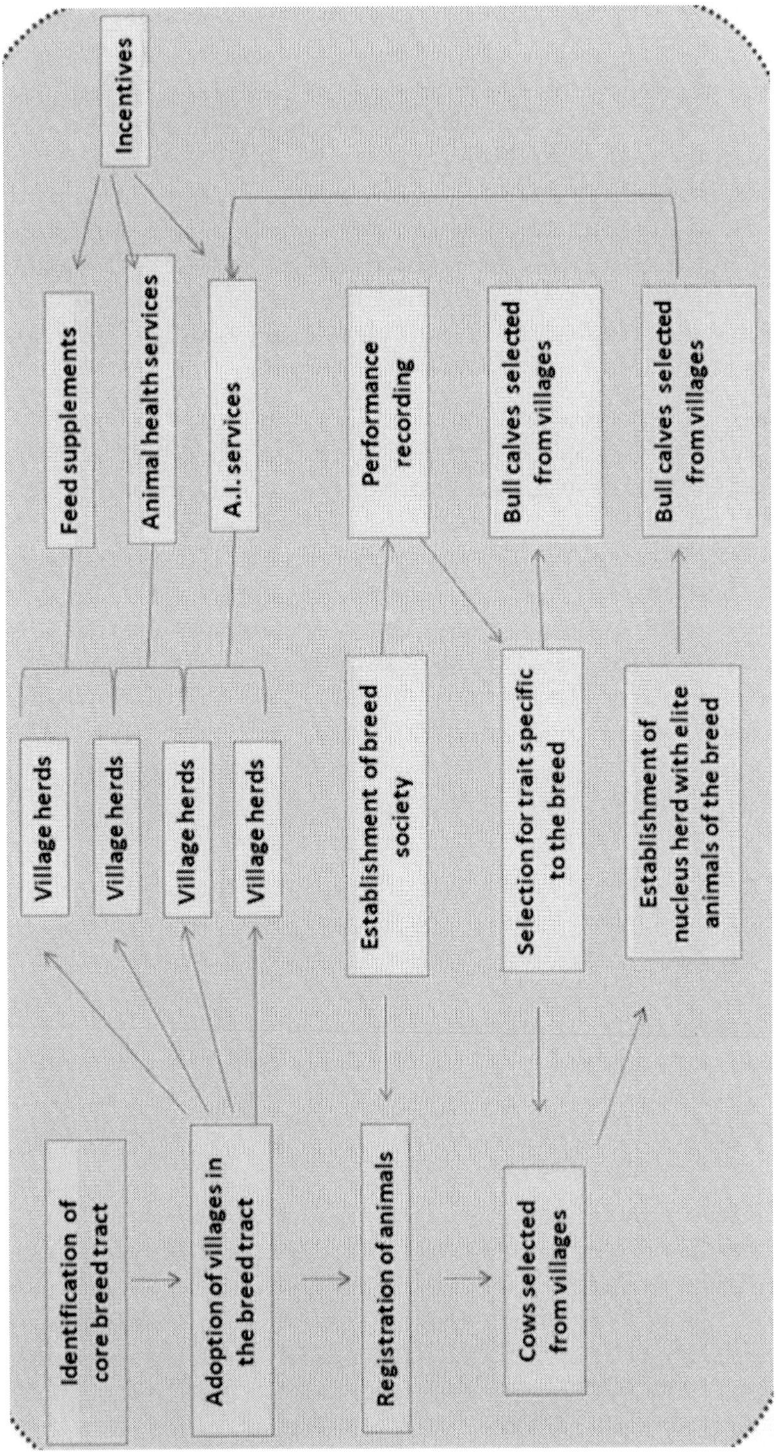

Figure 10.3 *In situ* conservation model involving farmers

Sustainable conservation of animal breeds with participation of farmers will be successful only if it is economically viable. Hence, the projects on conservation for improvement and utilization of breeds should define their objectives clearly especially with respect to those characteristics which the breed has been traditionally valued. The conservation efforts should begin with characterization and evaluation of breeds and identification of characteristics of economic/social/cultural significance specific to each breed. With the background information on the breed to be conserved, the nucleus area of native tract should be identified for adoption of selected villages to implement the conservation and improvement programme.

Breed society: Two to three villages belonging to each of five or six blocks distributed in different parts of the breed tract should be identified for the purpose. As a first step, the farmers and stakeholders should be motivated and facilitated to establish a breed society. The farmers who own animals true to the breed should be encouraged to register their animals with the society. The government support to the conservation program should be in the form of establishing a nucleus herd of the breed, field recording system and provision of certain services to the farmers. Breeding services like artificial insemination at farmers' doorstep, animal health services and feed supplements may be provided either free of cost or at subsidized rates.

A nucleus herd of 200 cows with at least 10-20 breedable males should be established in the breeding tract of the breed. An open nucleus breeding system should be followed with bi-directional gene flow from farm to field and vice versa. For a nucleus herd of 200 cows, the best 20 females may be selected from the villages each year as replacements for the animals to be culled from the nucleus herd. The same should be followed for breedable males also by replacing bulls in the herd with bull calves from the field. However, an efficient field recording system should be in place to identify the elite animals as well as to monitor the genetic improvement.

The breed society of the farmers should be made to actively participate in promoting and creating a brand for specific products derived from the breed conserved. Such measures will strength the economic value of the animals which can ultimately lead to its self-sustenance. In such case, the external support from the government can be gradually withdrawn while allowing the breed society to take over and continue the efforts in this direction.

10.6 Role of NGOs in breed conservation

Reputed NGOs may be involved in the conservation programmes after developing suitable MoU with them. Such organization may be financially supported only after developing a technical programme and targets to be achieved under the programmes.

10.7 Research and development organizations

Many R & D organizations like IVRI, NDRI, NBAGR, NDDB, Institute cattle breeding farms and state government breeding units should plan a common collaborative long term conservation research project for indigenous genetic resources. At present, these institutions are working independently with a technical programme for a specified period. The main drawback of such programmes is that after completing its technical programmes, there is no follow up mechanism from the state development agencies. Therefore, it is important that when the breed gets the status of 'Not at risk' after running the R&D programmes, the respective state government should develop some continuous activity for the breed so that their population size may be maintained or further increased.

10.8 Breed societies / Breeders' organizations

The Farmers should also be encouraged for establishing breed societies so as to provide better marketing and input facilities to animal keepers. Initially the Animal keepers should be supported financially and technically for establishing such institutions but after a certain period such societies should reach to a position of self-reliance. The Societies should be in the hands of the Animal keepers under a democratic way without any political or government interventions. The government, industrialists and politicians should support them as and when needed.

10.9 Conservation strategy for endangered breeds

It is possible now to store a wide variety of living cells for long periods of time. There is an urgent need to establish national level **Indigenous Cattle Cell Bank** where sperm, oocytes, embryos, DNA and embryonic stem cell should be conserved.

10.9.1 *Ex situ in-vivo conservation*

This implies keeping animals (often a very limited number) outside their natural habitat, so that natural selection is no longer effective in its role to assure adaptation of the population to its original environmental challenges. It is strongly advised to combine this method with cryoconservation. If reconstruction of a population with frozen semen is required, it might be very helpful to use the few purebred *ex situ in vivo* conserved females as founders, with semen from equal number of males.

10.9.2 *National live animal gene banks*

The institutional herds need to be strengthened both in terms of superior germplasm as well as modern tools and techniques. It is better if these farms are open nucleus herds rather than closed. There is a need to earmark at least one Livestock Farm to each of the breeds with fixed herd strength. These farms should be given mandate of conservation as well as genetic improvement of the breed. Following should be objectives of the farm:

a) To act as live animal gene bank for that breed.

b) To supply desired number of breeding stock to the farmers.

c) To act as demonstration unit for the farmers/take up extension activities i.e. capacity building at grass-root level.

10.10 *Ex situ in-vitro* conservation (cryopreservation)

Once the decision has been taken as to which breeds and populations should be there for the gene bank and the type of germplasm to be collect, the next step is to determine the amount of germplasm needed. The quantity will vary depending on the conservation goal, the type of germplasm and the species. In general, the goal of reconstituting extinct populations will require the greatest amount of germplasm.

Two criteria may be taken up to prioritize the breed for ex-situ conservation:

i) **Status of breed population**: Endangered/threatened should be taken first.

ii) **Economic contribution/unique traits in the breed.**

Material for cryoconservation (gametes, embryos) must meet high sanitary requirements and animal disease might disturb or inhibit collection of this material. Freezing, maintenance and thawing of frozen material require special skills and reliable equipments and infrastructures. To avoid risk, professional gene banks often store the material of an individual animal at two different locations.

a) Gene Bank

Gene bank is a place for storage of germplasm, provided that the germplasm is provided from elsewhere. Types and quantities of germplasm for a range of species and breeds to be placed in gene bank will decide the size and capacity of the banks, and similarly different equipments needed for the storage operation. Germplasm should be collected under highly sanitary conditions. Specialized work force as well as security of gene bank is also important.

Gene bank should be sufficiently large to store different types of germplasm. Gene bank should contain separate places for each activity like germplasm acquisition or collection, processing of germplasm and cryopreservation. The actual collection and banking of animal germplasm comprises of three main activities; collection processing and freezing and storage of the germplasm. All three activities require their own facilities. In most situations, a gene bank should have the infrastructure for at least two, if not all three activities.

b) Germplasm Collection Facility

It becomes more convenient when sufficient germplasm is to be collected in multiple interventions. Genebank may have separate central facility for such type of activities like semen and embryo collection. Donors should be kept in different buildings and follow all in/all out policy. Group of animals can be brought into empty and sanitized building and then animals should be quarantined and germplasm should be collected. Proper ventilation and humidity is essential in such animal sections. Air should flow from one direction in building so that least contamination will occur. Biosecurity is most important in animal section.

Collection of germplasm in field is practicable when a large number of breeds are distributed in similarly large geographical area. Field collection requires specific protocols to be followed as well as specialized equipment. Protocols related to collection from field should be followed as per FAO guidelines (FAO cryopreservation). Germplasm collected from field should be transferred in liquid nitrogen as early as possible. Biosecurity protocols should be followed to prevent the transmission of diseases from one location to another. The processing and freezing laboratories may be part of the same physical structure as the animal collection and holding facilities but there should be a distinct physical barrier between the two areas as the processing and freezing area must have a greater level of sanitation. The laboratory should be designed for maximum efficiency. In particular, it should be kept as small as possible to decrease the area to maintain and keep clean and the various workstations should be arranged in a logical order so that germplasm samples more in a progressive order from workstation to workstation.

c) Regional Semen Bank

The State Livestock Development Boards may also establish Regional Semen banks. The Conservation Advisory body will decide the priority of breeds for conservation. State Livestock Development Boards may supervise the Frozen Semen Production Units in the state and the activity of breeding of field animals (AI Centres).

d) Collection of germplasm and tissue

The type of genetic resource material to be preserved in the gene bank depends on the purpose of the gene bank. Genrally gene bank concept is intended to preserve the germplasm for *ex situ in vitro* conservation strategy to save and preserve present day biodiversity for "eternity" or at least for improbable emergency situations in the finite future. For long term conservation programme, fast collection of various type of germplasm from all indigenous cattle breeds as possible is needed. Still, semen is the best choice for such strategy, when there are financial constraints and we have to make the collection very fast. It needs simple techniques and expertise. However, wherever financial resources and existing expertise and facilities are available, embryos are probably the best choice, but in lack of that, collection and cryopreservation of somatic cells could be considered as a possibility.

It is also important to duplicate the material and store the sets of samples at separate locations in order to reduce risks of loss. Conserve small amounts of germplasm from many donor animals rather than large amounts from few donors. Choose donors that are as genetically and phenotypically diverse as possible; and store the breeds as pure lines rather than gene pools, so as to allow the use of the unique combinations of traits and flexibility in the combination of stocks.

e) Semen

Semen is widely used germplasm for livestock improvement programmes as well as cryopreservation. Almost in all livestock species, this technique has been standardized. It can be stored easily and reused for reconstitution of a individual or population through backcrossing. Well equipped infrastructure for semen collection across the country makes it easiest way for germplasm storage. Banking of sexed semen may potentially decrease the number of doses required for storage.

f) Embryos

Embryos are one of the best germplasm, as an option to reconstitute any breed/species in faster way. Birth from cryopreserved embryo has been achieved in almost all the livestock species. When technology for the collection and preservation of embryos for a species is available, it is the best option for conserving genetic diversity. However, it is more costly and requires advanced technologies for collection and preservation. At present, embryo cryopreservation for cattle is highly efficient.

g) DNA bank

Genetic material of all the indigenous breeds can be preserved in the form of DNA fragments under cryogenic conditions. This has the advantage over storage of live cells as it is economical, occupies less space and there is no spread of diseases. Although it is easiest method for preservation, however, at present, DNA is not used for recreating the live animals. However, at the same time, it is useful in characterization and development of breed signatures of indigenous cattle breeds and support conservation decision.

h) Online inventory of germplasm

All the germplasm should be maintained through proper online record system. There should be set format for the information needed for proper identification. Details about donor, its pedigree, index score, physical characters, production record (for female or sire's dam), physical traits, disease etc. Photograph of the animal should also be taken. Similarly quality of germplasm should also be recorded and maintained in proper inventory from time to time. Inventories for each type of germplasm should be separate.

i) Quality control

Quality of frozen semen stored in Gene Bank is an important issue and must be taken care seriously and regularly. The breeding males should be regularly identified for important communicable diseases like Brucellosis, Vibriosis, Trichomoniasis. The details of bull pedigree, physical characteristics and bull's semen quality should also be supplied by cooperating centers for documenting the details of frozen semen stored in Gene Bank. The semen doses should have the microbial load within the permissible limits.

The recommendations for collection, treatment and storage of embryos/oocytes and semen are based on OIE recommendations and other sources. The regulations at international level (OIE, International Embryo Transfer Society), of recommendations, which, each country, is free to follow or not.

The breeding soundness of bulls to be used for semen collection, the disease screening and other protocols for semen collection has to be followed as per the international guidelines by FAO and OIE (World Organization for Animal Health). There are no existences, however, of any regulation for somatic cells and DNA. In general, the collected material, collection and treatment must comply with veterinary rules. It is important to categorize the genetic material to be cryopreserved in terms of compliance with regulations. Several categories can be established. A regular examination of the semen kept at National and Regional Gene Banks may be carried out so as to the fertility status of semen doses.

❑❑❑

CHAPTER-11

Gau Sanrakshan and Samvardhan through Women Empowerment

In India, 70% of the rural households own livestock. They are an important source of employment in rural India, especially for women. In spite of the fact that the average holding of livestock is small, the livestock sector has considerable potential for generating additional employment through milk, meat, wool and eggs production. Milk production alone involves more than 30 million small producers.

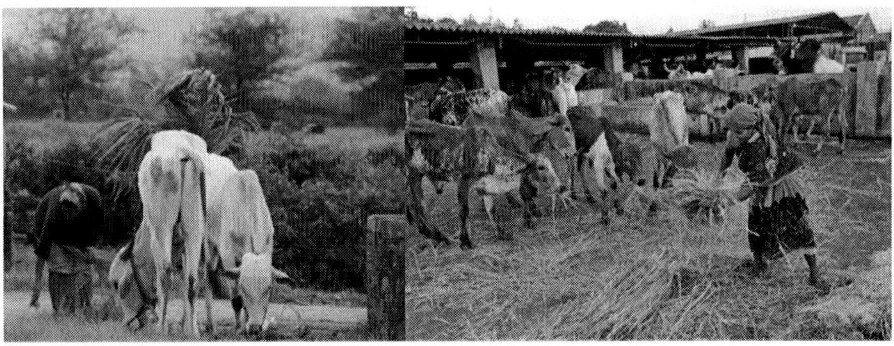

Gender equality is more pronounced in livestock sector, as women participation is 71% of the labour force while it is only 33% in crop farming. As many as 75 million women are engaged in the livestock sector as against 15 million men. Women play a major role in livestock production and most of them have good knowledge about livestock behavior and local feeds. Extent and nature of their involvement varies within and between regions. Despite variations, women mostly handle aspects like milking, care of young and sick animals, cleaning and feeding.

Livestock sector empowers women as they perform a large number of activities related to livestock production. According to the working group report on animal husbandry and dairying 12th five year plan (2012-17), animal husbandry helps in improving gender equity. More than three-fourth of the labour requirement in livestock production is met by women. The share of women employment in livestock sector is around 90% in Punjab and Haryana where dairying is a major activity. The outstanding demand for livestock products gives considerable opportunities for the rural women to escape poverty by diversifying livestock production. Animal husbandry provides large self employment opportunities to rural females in India. In fact animal husbandry is becoming more and more feminized. Animal husbandry is the second most important agricultural activity after cultivation in providing self-employment to rural women while it is the main source of self-employment to them, among non-crop activities. Thus, government must promote investment in this sector to enhance self-employment among rural people. Animal husbandry is the only agricultural activity among all agricultural activities which has increased the casual, regular and self-employment to female. Animal husbandry is again the only agricultural activity which is making women more self-employed than men. Thus, livestock enterprise is more women oriented and growth in this sector would help in promoting gender equity and empowerment of women in rural India. Development of this sector can become instrumental in empowering women by providing them large self-employment opportunities.

Women play an important role in livestock related activities, yet they face various challenges than men in accessing natural resources, market opportunities, extension services, technology, credit, information, inputs and services, etc. It is difficult for them to reach their full potential in agricultural sector including livestock sector. Following suggestions can be given to take advantage of the opportunities given this booming sector to empower rural women:

a) Policy makers should seriously recognize the women's role in livestock sector. Women should be incorporated in overall development process like more women should be employed in dairy extension and other kinds of dissemination work and in policy making as well.

b) Proper education is a very important factor. Women should be educated about the opportunity in the growing livestock sector of India to become an entrepreneur or a worker in the growing industry.

c) Unfortunately curriculum in agricultural/Veterinary universities does not give importance to gender issues. Gender issues must be covered under the curriculum in agricultural/Veterinary universities to make more gender sensitive policies and programmes in dairy sector.

d) Rural women should be given enough access to financial, extension services, new technologies and markets so that her potential can be optimized.

e) Women livestock workers form a heterogeneous group so the policy framed for the whole country may prove ineffective when there are distinct differences among rural women based on caste, geographical area, type of livestock reared and livestock products.

❑❑❑

CHAPTER-12

Human Cow Bonding

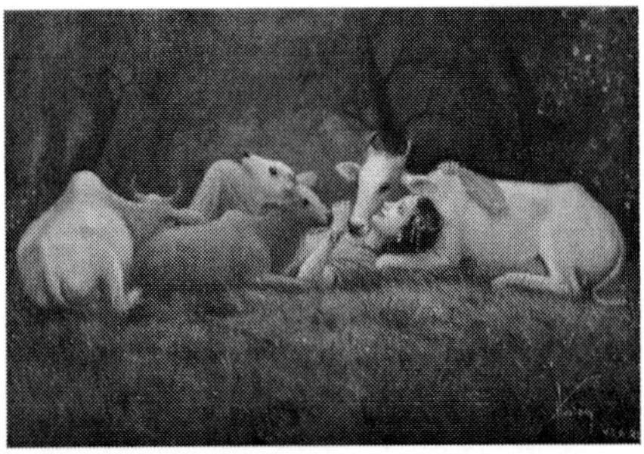

Cows and Krishna have always been together. In His original form in the spiritual world, Krishna is a cow herd boy in the agricultural community of Goloka ("cow planet") Vrindavan, where He keeps unlimited, transcendental surabhi cows. When He descends to earth, Krishna brings a replica of Vrindavan with Him, and He spends His childhood tending cows and calves while playing in the pasturing grounds with his friends. His example shows the importance of cows to human society, the practical benefits of caring for them, and the advantages of an agrarian economy based on cooperation between man and cows.

Krishna is also known as Govinda "He who gives pleasure to cows". Krishna established the original economic system, varnashrama-dharma, for the spiritual and material progress of all living beings. Protected cows are a major component of this system; bulls and oxen till the fields, and cows give milk. Cows are considered one of the mothers of humankind because cow's milk—when properly prepared—is perfectly suited to maintaining human life. Milk can be made into a wide variety of preparations, such as yogurt and butter, which are also essential ingredients for use in the ceremonial worship of Krishna in His transcendental Deity form.

In His famous book of instructions for humankind, the Bhagavad-Gita, Krishna mentions cow protection as one of the prime duties of any civilized society. The Bible also tells us that cow-killing is as punishable as killing a human being.

12.1 Scientific vision to Govinda

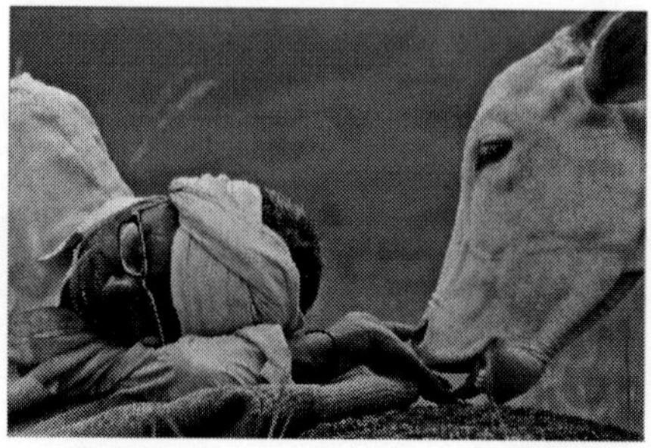

Many studies conducted globally indicated that the variation in milk production among dairies was due to cow handling and reported a significant relationships between the behavioral response to humans and the milk production of cows. Cow behaviors that are indicative of fear of humans were moderately or highly correlated with milk yield and composition.

Many researchers reported that where restlessness was high, productivity was low and animal was more prone to disease. Animal handling and understanding their feeling is not a child play and it's a totally neglected area. Sympathetic and protective environment must be provided for overall well being and harvesting the milk yield.

Therefore, there is an urgent need to intiate a long term project on "Cattle behavior genetics decoding" at national level to rediscover the behavioral genetics of our indigenous cows to increase productivity.

□□□

CHAPTER-13

Important Rules for Conservation

a) Every breeding animal must be replaced by his/her progeny.

b) Strict parental verification procedure must be adopted (DFD marker).

c) The percentage of the known or visible characteristics must be kept approximately around the foundation frequency.

d) Possibly also the immunogenetic characteristics should be used.

e) The generation interval must be kept as long as possible according to breed or species.

f) The number of males in consecutive years must be as many as possible.

13.1 Essential considerations for conservation

a) Judicious and scientific management of livestock breeds.

b) Strategies for the preservation of less productive breeds with adequate genetic variability and distinct characteristics.

c) Alternate use/value addition of products of the breed.

d) Establishment of the *in situ* and *ex situ* gene banks.

e) Establishment of informatics and computation system with data banks and interactive networking with other global agencies.

f) Setting up Livestock Conservation Boards.

g) Formulation of well defined breeding policies consistent both with conservation and economic situations of the farmers.

h) Formulation of livestock population policy consistent with the carrying capacity and environmental management.

i) People participation through Breed societies, Associations, Breed survival trusts and NGO's.

j) Setting modalities for gene banks, data banks and genetic resource movement/transfer.

k) Development of financial and institutional mechanism for conservation programmes.

13.2 Problems faced in conservation approaches

a) There continues to be pronounced general dearth of information on animal genetic resources.

b) Fragmentation of land holding and preponderance of small number of animals with location in remote rural areas.

c) Virtual non-existence of breed registration societies for operation of pedigree/performance recording programme and breed characterization work. Genus data are not maintained breed wise and more often are not reliable.

d) No proper tie up of livestock development programmes with problems of conservation, management and evaluation of genetic resources and their utilization.

e) There should be a balance between conservation goal and resource utilization.

f) Incredible pressure of human population has produced conflict situations and problems due to variety of interactions between people and our natural environment.

g) All important monetary resources crunch can create problems of un-imaginable proportions.

13.3 Stakeholders for conservation of indigenous cattle

a) Government Institutions /Research organizations

b) Livestock keepers, owners, breeders, pastoralists and users

c) Non Governmental Organizations/Gaushalas

d) Breed associations, Societies

e) Breeding companies

f) Product processing and marketing agencies

g) Consumers/Consumer bodies using the breed's products

□□□

References

A. Cieslinska, S. Kamiñski, E. Kostyra and E. Sienkiewicz-Szlapka (2007), Betacasomorphin7 in raw and hydrolyzed milk derived from cows of alternative β-casein genotypes, *Milchwissenschaft*, 62: 125-127.

Basic Animal Husbandry Statistics (2014), DAHD&F, Ministry of Animal Husbandry, Dairying and Fisheries, Ministry of Agriculture, Government of India, India.

Basic Animal Husbandry Statistics (2015), DAHD&F, Ministry of Animal Husbandry, Dairying and Fisheries, Ministry of Agriculture, Government of India, India.

Breed survey report (2013), DAHD&F, Ministry of Animal Husbandry, Dairying and Fisheries, Ministry of Agriculture, Government of India, India.

C.N. McLachlan (2001), Beta-casein A1, ischaemic heart disease mortality, and other illnesses, *Med. Hypotheses*, 56: 262–272.

De Noni I. (2008), Release of β-casomorphins 5 and 7 during simulated gastro-intestinal digestion of bovine β-casein variants and milk-based infant formulas. *Food Chemistry* 110: 897-903.

Farrell, H.M., Jimenez-Flores, R., Bleck, G.T., Brown, E.M., Butler, J.E. & Creamer, L.K. (2004), Nomenclature of the proteins of cows' milk - sixth revision. *J. Dairy Sci., Vol.* 87: 1641-1674.

H. Roginski (2003), Encyclopedia of dairy sciences, Academic Press, London.

K.A. Tailford, C.L. Berry, A.C. Thomas and J.H. Campbell (2003), A casein variant in cow's milk is atherogenic, *Atherosclerosis,* 170: 13–19.

M. Laugesen and R. Elliott (2003), Ischaemic heart disease, type 1 diabetes, and cow milk A1 beta-casein. *New. Zeal. Med. J,* 116: 1–19.

National Programme for Prevention and Control of Cancer, Diabetes, Cardiovascular Diseases and Stroke report. (2013), (NPCDCS), Ministry of Health and Welfare, Government of India.

R.B. Elliott, D.P. Harris, J.P. Hill, N.J. Bibby and H.E. Wasmuth, (1999), Type I (insulindependent) diabetes mellitus and cow milk: casein variant consumption, *Diabetologia* 42: 292–296.

Z. Sun, Z. Zhang, X. Wang, R. Cade, Z. Elmer and M Fregly (2003), Relation of beta-casomorphin to apnea in sudden infant death syndrome, *Peptides*, 24: 937–943.

18th livestock Census (2007), All India Report, Department of Animal Husbandry, Dairying and Fisheries, Ministry of Agriculture, Government of India.

19th livestock Census (2012), All India Report, Department of Animal Husbandry, Dairying and Fisheries, Ministry of Agriculture, Government of India.

http://www.nbagr.res.in/contact.html

http://cowbank.in/index.php/2014-07-14-05-27-20.

□□□